Place $2\frac{7}{8} \times 2\frac{7}{8}$ **Sticky Notes** here
for a convenient and refillable note pad

HIPAA compliant
OSHA compliant

D0154573

Waterproof and Reusable
Wipe-Free Pages

Write directly onto any page of *Phlebotomy Notes*
with a ballpoint pen. Wipe old entries off with an
alcohol pad and reuse.

| EQUIP | VENI PUNCT | COMPLI-CATIONS | SPECIAL PROC | DERMAL PUNCT | ARTERIAL PUNCT | SAFETY | LABS |

Equipment

Evacuated Tube System
BD Vacutainer Venous Blood
  Collection Tube Guide
Vacuette Tube Guide
CLSI Recommended Order of
  Draw
Common Tests Affected by
  Additive Carryover
Syringe System
Winged Blood Collection Sets
Additional Equipment
Equipment Quality Control

Venipuncture

Common Venipuncture Veins
Patient Identification
Patient Positioning
Tourniquet Application
Palpating the Vein
Anchoring the Vein
Venipuncture Using an ETS
Venipuncture Using a Syringe
Venipuncture Using a Winged
  Blood Collection Set

Venipuncture Complications

Major Tests Affected by Patient
  Pre-examination Variables
Effects of Medications on
  Laboratory Tests
Failure to Obtain Blood
Patient Complications
Technical Errors Affecting the
  Patient
Technical Errors Affecting the
  Specimen
Laboratory Tests Affected by
  Hemolysis

Special Procedures

Timed Specimens
Blood Cultures

Special Specimen Handling
  Procedures
Blood Collection From Vascular
  Access Devices
Urine Collection
Throat Culture Collection
Point of Care Testing (POCT)

Dermal Puncture

Dermal Puncture Sites
Dermal Puncture Procedure
Order of Draw Using BD
  Microtainer Tubes
Newborn Screening
Capillary Blood Gas Collection
  by Heel Puncture
Preparation of Blood Smears

Arterial Puncture

Arterial Blood Collection
Arterial Blood Gas Tests
Specimen Integrity
Effects of Technical Errors on
  ABG Result
Arterial Puncture Complications

Safety

Infection Control
Personal Immunization
  Information
Transmission-Based Precautions
  Classifications
Sharps Precautions
Chemical Precautions
Radiation Precautions
Electrical Precautions
Fire and Explosion Precautions
Physical Precautions
Location of Safety Equipment

Laboratory Tests

Common Laboratory Tests and
  Collection Tube Requirements

References

Resources and References

2nd Edition

Phlebotomy
Notes

Pocket Guide to Blood Collection

Susan King Strasinger,
DA, MT (ASCP)

Marjorie Schaub Di Lorenzo
MT (ASCP), SH

Purchase additional copies of this book at your health science bookstore or directly from F.A. Davis by shopping online at www.fadavis.com or by calling 800-323-3555 (US) or 800-665-1148 (CAN)

A Davis's Notes Book

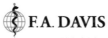

F.A. DAVIS

Philadelphia

F.A. Davis Company

1915 Arch Street
Philadelphia, PA 19103
www.fadavis.com

Copyright © 2020 by F.A. Davis Company

Printed in China

Last digit indicates print number: 10 9 8 7 6 5 4 3

Senior Acquisitions Editor: Christa Fratantoro
Director of Content Development: George W. Lang
Senior Developmental Editor: Dean W. DeChambeau
Content Project Manager: Megan Suermann
Design and Illustration Manager: Carolyn O'Brien

All of the photographs and several of the illustrations included in this product are adapted from Strasinger, SK and Di Lorenzo, MS: *The Phlebotomy Textbook*, ed. 4. FA Davis, 2019, Philadelphia, with permission.

As new scientific information becomes available through basic and clinical research, recommended treatments and drug therapies undergo changes. The author(s) and publisher have done everything possible to make this book accurate, up to date, and in accord with accepted standards at the time of publication. The author(s), editors, and publisher are not responsible for errors or omissions or for consequences from application of the book, and make no warranty, expressed or implied, in regard to the contents of the book. Any practice described in this book should be applied by the reader in accordance with professional standards of care used in regard to the unique circumstances that may apply in each situation. The reader is advised always to check product information (package inserts) for changes and new information regarding dose and contraindications before administering any drug. Caution is especially urged when using new or infrequently ordered drugs.

Evacuated Tube System

An evacuated tube system (ETS) consists of:

- Double-pointed multisample needle
  - One point to puncture the stopper of the collection tube
  - One point to puncture the patient's vein
- Needle safety device
- Holder to hold the needle and the collection tube
- Color-coded evacuated tubes

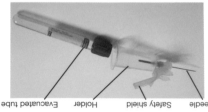

Needle — Safety shield — Holder — Evacuated tube

Needles

Needle size varies by length and gauge and is indicated by color-coded caps. Gauge refers to the needle's diameter: the lower the number, the larger the needle.

Standard Sizes

- Routine venipuncture: 21- or 22-gauge with 1- or 1.5-inch length
- Children and patients with small veins: 22- or 23-gauge with ³/₄-inch length

💧 **ALERT:** Use of a 25-gauge needle is not recommended because the needle must remain in the vein longer, increasing the likelihood of hemolysis and clotting.

✋ **ALERT**: Use of a 20-gauge needle can result in postpuncture bleeding and hematomas for patients who are taking blood thinners.

Needle Safety Features

- Provide containment of needle after use.
- Must be activated with one hand.

✋ **ALERT**: The blood collector must keep his or her hand behind the needle at all times.

Types of Safety Devices

- Safety shield: Locks over the needle.

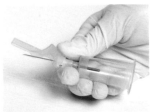

- Blunting device: Causes the needle to blunt before removal from the vein.
- In-vein retraction device: Automatically activates to retract the needle while it is still in the patient's vein.

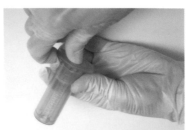

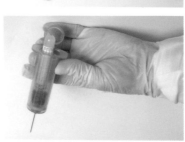

✋ **ALERT:** According to OSHA regulations, if a needle does not have a safety device, the tube holder or syringe must have a safety device to prevent accidental needlesticks.

Holders

Holders are available with and without safety features.

Assembly

- Screw the stopper-puncturing end of the ETS needle into the holder.
- Advance the blood collection tube on to the stopper-puncturing needle up to the tube advancement mark.
- Fully advance the tube to the end of the holder when the needle is in the vein.

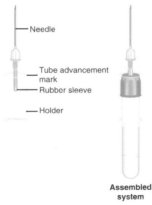

— Needle

— Tube advancement mark
— Rubber sleeve

— Holder

Assembled system

✋ **ALERT**: Do not push the needle beyond the designated mark on the holder before inserting the needle into the vein. Doing so breaks the tube's vacuum, making the tube unusable.

Test	Collection Tube	Comments	Dept.
Vitamin B_6	Green	No gel barrier tubes; ensure patient has fasted; protect from light	C
Vitamin B_{12}	Plasma (green) or serum (red or gold) gel barrier tube; red	Protect from light	C
Vitamin D	Serum (red or gold) gel barrier tube		C
Western blot	Red		I
White blood cell (WBC) count	Lavender		H
Zinc	Plain royal blue; lime green		C

Lab department codes: BB = blood bank; C = chemistry; CO = coagulation; H = hematology; I = immunology; M = microbiology; ID = identification; RT = room temperature; SPS = sodium polyanethol sulfonate.
Follow evacuated tube manufacturer's instructions when using gel barrier tubes for immunology tests.
Follow facility protocol for placing specimens in an ice slurry.
Collection tube requirements may vary among facilities depending on the instrument used and the test methodology.

Resources and References

Useful Web Sites

- American Society for Clinical Pathology: www.ascp.org
- Becton, Dickinson and Company: www.bd.com
- Center for Phlebotomy Education: www.phlebotomy.com
- Centers for Disease Control and Prevention: www.cdc.gov
- Clinical and Laboratory Standards Institute (CLSI): www.clsi.org
- Greiner Bio-One: www.gbo.com
- Lab Tests Online: www.labtestsonline.org
- Occupational Safety and Health Administration: www.osha.gov

References

CLSI. Accuracy in Patient and Sample Identification. Approved Guideline GP33-A. Clinical and Laboratory Standards Institute, Wayne, PA, 2010.

CLSI. Blood Collection on Filter Paper for Newborn Screening Programs. Approved Standard, ed. 6. CLSI document NBS01-A6. Clinical and Laboratory Standards Institute, Wayne, PA, 2013.

CLSI. Collection of Diagnostic Venous Blood Specimens, ed. 7. CLSI standard GP41. Clinical and Laboratory Standards Institute, Wayne, PA, 2017.

CLSI. Collection, Transport, and Processing of Blood Specimens for Testing Plasma-Based Coagulation Assays and Molecular Hemostasis Assays. Approved Guideline, ed. 5. CLSI document H21-A5. Clinical and Laboratory Standards Institute, Wayne, PA, 2008.

CLSI. Procedures for the Collection of Arterial Blood Specimens. Approved Standard, ed. 4. CLSI document GP43-A4. Clinical and Laboratory Standards Institute, Wayne, PA, 2004.

CLSI. Procedures and Devices for the Collection of Diagnostic Capillary Blood Specimens. Approved Standard, ed. 6. CLSI

5

NEEDLE AND SHARPS DISPOSAL CONTAINERS

Dispose of used needles, lancets, and other sharp objects in sharps disposal containers. Containers must be:

- Labeled "biohazard"
- Rigid, puncture-resistant, and leakproof
- Equipped with locking lids

Seal the container when the appropriate volume "fill" line is reached.

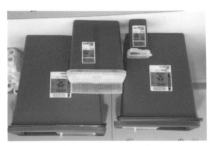 **ALERT:** Do not overfill a sharps container.

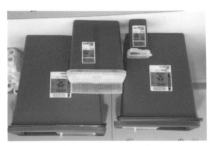 **ALERT:** Never recap a needle under any circumstance.

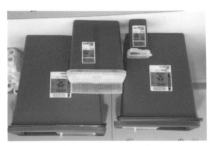

Collection Tubes

Evacuated tubes are labeled with:

- Type of anticoagulant or other additive indicated by the color-coded stopper
- Draw volume
- Expiration date
- Lot number

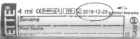

Additives

Anticoagulants

Tests requiring whole blood or plasma are collected in tubes containing an anticoagulant to prevent clotting of the specimen by:

- Binding or chelating calcium
  - EDTA
  - Citrates
  - Oxalates
- Inhibiting thrombin
  - Heparin

ALERT: Do not transfer blood collected in a tube containing an anticoagulant or other type of additive into a tube containing a different anticoagulant or additive.

Anticoagulants With Preservatives

- Acid citrate dextrose (ACD): Preserves RBC viability
- Sodium polyanethol sulfonate (SPS): Inhibits complement, phagocytes, and certain antibiotics

Antiglycolytic
- Sodium fluoride: Preserves glucose and inhibits bacterial growth

Clot Activators
- Silica: Increases platelet activation
- Thrombin: Promotes clotting

Polymer Barrier Gel
- Forms a barrier between the cells and serum or plasma after centrifugation

✋ **ALERT:** For anticoagulants and additives to be totally effective, specimens must be thoroughly mixed three to eight times immediately after collection.

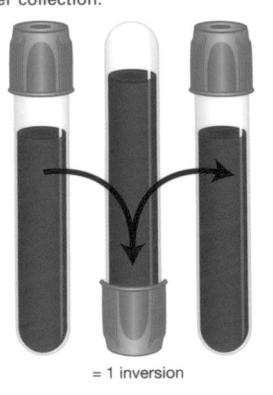

= 1 inversion

BD Vacutainer Venous Blood Collection Tube Guide

Hemogard™ Closure	Conventional Stopper	Additive	Inv	Laboratory Use	Notes
Gold	Red/Gray	• Clot activator and gel for serum separation	5	For serum determinations in chemistry. Blood clotting time: 30 minutes.	
Light Green	Green/Gray	• Lithium heparin and gel for plasma separation	8	For plasma determinations in chemistry.	
Red	Red	• Silicone coated (glass) • Clot activator, silicone coated (plastic)	0 / 5	For serum determinations in chemistry. Blood clotting time glass: 60 minutes. Blood clotting time, plastic: 30 minutes.	
Orange	Orange	• Thrombin-based clot activator with gel for serum separation	5 to 6	For stat serum determinations in chemistry. Blood clotting time: 5 minutes.	
Orange	Orange	• Thrombin-based clot activator	8	For stat serum determinations in chemistry. Blood clotting time: 5 minutes.	

*Inversions at blood collection

Hemogard™ Closure	Conventional Stopper	Additive	Inv	Laboratory Use	Notes
Royal Blue		• Clot activator (plastic serum) • K_2EDTA (plastic)	5 8	For trace-element, toxicology, and nutritional-chemistry determinations.	
Green	Green	• Sodium heparin • Lithium heparin	8 8	For plasma determinations in chemistry.	
Gray	Gray	• Potassium oxalate/ sodium fluoride • Sodium fluoride/ Na_2 EDTA • Sodium fluoride (serum tube)	8 8 8	For glucose determinations.	
Tan		• K_2EDTA (plastic)	8	For lead determinations.	
Lavender	Lavender	• Liquid K_3EDTA (glass) • Spray-coated K_2EDTA (plastic)	8 8	For whole blood hematology determinations.	

*Inversions at blood collection

Hemogard™ Closure	Conventional Stopper	Additive	Inv	Laboratory Use	Notes
	Yellow	• Sodium polyanethol sulfonate (SPS)	8	SPS for blood culture specimens in microbiology.	
		• Acid citrate dextrose additives (ACD): **Solution A** 22.0 g/L trisodium citrate, 8.0 g/L citric acid, 24.5 g/L dextrose **Solution B** 13.2 g/L trisodium citrate, 4.8 g/L citric acid, 14.7 g/L dextrose	8 8	ACD for blood bank studies, HLA phenotyping, and DNA and paternity testing.	
White		• K₂EDTA and gel for plasma separation	8	For use in molecular diagnostic test methods.	
Pink	Pink	• Spray-coated K₂EDTA (plastic)	8	For whole blood immunohematology testing. Special cross-match label.	

*inversions at blood collection

Hemogard™ Closure	Conventional Stopper	Additive	Inv	Laboratory Use	Notes
Light Blue	Light Blue	• Buffered sodium citrate 0.105 M (≈3.2%) glass 0.109 M (3.2%) plastic • Citrate, theophylline, adenosine, dipyridamole (CTAD)	3–4 3–4	For coagulation determinations.	
Clear	Light Blue				
Clear	Red/ Light Gray	• None (plastic)	0	For use as a discard tube or secondary specimen tube.	

*Inversions at blood collection

Courtesy of © Becton, Dickinson and Company. Adapted with permission.

Vacuette Tube Guide

Cap Colors	Additive	Number of Inversions	Testing Disciplines
	No additive*	5–10	Discard tube Transport/Storage Immunohematology Viral Markers
	Sodium Citrate 3.2% (0.109 M*)	4	Coagulation
	Clot Activator*	5–10	Chemistry Immunochemistry Immunohematology Viral Markers
	Clot Activator w/Gel	5–10	Chemistry Immunochemistry TDMs
	Lithium Heparin* Lithium Heparin w/Gel Sodium Heparin*	5–10	Chemistry Immunochemistry

Also available in pediatric or low draw volumes of 2mL or less.

Cap Colors	Additive	Number of Inversions	Testing Disciplines
	K EDTA* K EDTA*	8–10	Hematology Immunohematology Molecular Diagnostics Viral Markers
	K EDTA Gel	8–10	Molecular Diagnostics
	Potassium Oxalate/ Sodium Fluoride*	5–10	Glycolytic Inhibitor Glucose and Lactate
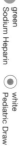	Sodium Heparin No Additive	5–10	Trace Elements

* Also available in pediatric or low draw volumes of 2mL or less.

- yellow
Gel Separation
- black
Standard Draw
- green
Sodium Heparin
- white
Pediatric Draw

Centrifugation Recommendations

Tube Type	G-Force	Minutes
VACUETTE® Serum Tubes (Clot Activator, No Additive)	Min. 1500 g	10
VACUETTE® Serum Clot Activator w/Gel Tubes	1800 g	10
VACUETTE® K₂EDTA w/Gel Tubes	1800–2200 g	10
VACUETTE® Plasma Tubes (Lithium or Sodium Heparin, PO/NaF)	2000–3000 g	15
VACUETTE® Lithium Heparin w/Gel Tubes	1800–2200 g	10–15
VACUETTE® Coagulation Tubes (Sodium Citrate)		
Platelet tests (PRP)	150 g	5
Routine tests (PPP)	1500–2000 g	10
Preparation for deep freeze plasma (PFP)	2530–3000 g	20

VACUETTE® Tube Guide. Courtesy of © Grenier Bio-One.

CLSI Recommended Order of Draw

Fill tubes in the following order to prevent invalid test results caused by contamination of the specimen by microorganisms, tissue thromboplastin, and additive carryover.

Order	Tube Color	Additive	Number of Inversions
1	Yellow	SPS Sterile media bottles	8–10
2	Light blue	Sodium citrate	3–4
3	Red plastic	Clot activator	5
	Red glass	No additive	0
	Red and gray SST	Gel separator tube with clot activator	5
	Gold SST	Gel separator tube with clot activator	5
	Orange RST	Gel separator tube with thrombin	5–6
	Royal blue	Clot activator	5–6
4	Light green PST	Gel separator tube with heparin	8–10
	Green	Heparin	
	Royal blue	Heparin	
5	Lavender	EDTA	8–10
	Pink	EDTA	
	Tan	EDTA	
	Royal blue	EDTA	
	White PPT	Gel separator with EDTA	
6	Gray	Potassium oxalate Sodium fluoride	8–10
7	Yellow	ACD	8–10

Courtesy of © Becton, Dickinson and Company. Adapted with permission.

✋ ALERT: Always follow your facility's protocol for order of draw.

Order of Draw Notes

_____

_____

_____

_____

_____

_____

_____

_____

_____

_____

_____

_____

_____

_____

_____

_____

_____

_____

_____

Common Tests Affected by Additive Carryover

Additive	Possible Compromised Test
Clot activator (silica)	• Activated partial thromboplastin time (APTT) • Prothrombin time (PT)
EDTA	• Acid phosphatase • Activated partial thromboplastin time • Alkaline phosphatase • Alpha-1-antitrypsin • Amylase • Calcium • Ceruloplasmin • Cholinesterase • Copper • Creatine kinase-MB (CK-MB) • Creatinine • Iron • Iron binding capacity • Lipase • Lipids • Potassium • Prothrombin time (PT) • Sodium • Uric acid
Heparin	• Acid phosphatase • Activated clotting time • APTT • Albumin • Ammonia (ammonium heparin) • Blood urea nitrogen (BUN) (ammonium heparin) • Cholinesterase • CK-MB

Continued

Additive	Possible Compromised Test
	• Erythrocyte sedimentation rate (ESR)
	• Gamma-glutamyl transferase (gamma-GT)
	• Iron
	• Lithium (lithium heparin)
	• PT
	• Sodium (sodium heparin)
Potassium oxalate	• Acid phosphatase
	• APTT
	• Alkaline phosphatase
	• Amylase
	• Bilirubin
	• Calcium
	• CK-MB
	• Copper
	• Creatine kinase (CK)
	• Gamma-GT
	• Insulin
	• Iron
	• Lactate dehydrogenase (LDH)
	• Lipid electrophoresis
	• Lithium
	• Low-density lipoprotein (LDL) cholesterol
	• Potassium
	• Protein electrophoresis
	• PT
	• Red blood cell morphology
	• Sodium
	• Triiodothyronine (T_3)
	• Triglycerides
	• Vitamin B_{12}
Sodium citrate	• Acid phosphatase
	• Alkaline phosphatase
	• Alpha-1-antitrypsin
	• Amylase
	• Bilirubin

Continued

Additive	Possible Compromised Test
	• Calcium • Cholesterol • CK-MB • Copper • Creatine kinase (CK) • Creatinine • Gamma-GT • Glucose • High-density lipoprotein (HDL) cholesterol • Iron • Phosphorus • Sodium • Triglycerides • Uric acid
Sodium fluoride	• Acid phosphatase • Alanine aminotransferase (ALT) • Alkaline phosphatase • Amylase • Aspartate aminotransferase (AST) • Bilirubin • BUN • Cholesterol • Cholinesterase • CK-MB • Copper • Creatine kinase (CK) • Creatinine • Gamma-GT • HDL cholesterol • LDH • Sodium • Triglycerides • Uric acid

Syringe System

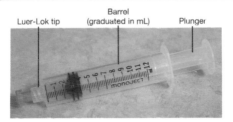

Luer-Lok tip | Barrel (graduated in mL) | Plunger

The syringe system consists of:

- Hypodermic needle with safety device
- Plastic syringe with a Luer-Lok tip

Uses
- Small, fragile veins
- Elderly patients
- Pediatric patients

Blood Transfer Device

A blood transfer device is used to transfer blood into ETS tubes. After the syringe draw is complete:

- Activate the needle safety device.
- Remove the needle and dispose of it in a sharps disposal container.
- Attach the transfer device to the hub of the syringe.
- Place the ETS tube inside the holder and advance it on to the rubber-sheathed stopper-puncturing needle until blood flows into the tube.
- Fill additional tubes according to the correct order of draw.

Winged Blood Collection Sets

A winged blood collection set consists of:

- 1/2- or 3/4-inch needle connected to 5- to 12-inch length of tubing
- Plastic wings that attach to the needle for a lower insertion angle
- Luer attachment for syringe use or evacuated tube holder

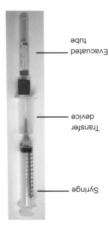

Syringe

Transfer device

Evacuated tube

ALERT: Hold the syringe, blood transfer device, and tube in a vertical position to prevent additive carryover.

ALERT: Do not push the plunger to force blood into the tube. Allow the vacuum in the evacuated tube to draw the correct amount of blood into the tube.

Uses
- Small, fragile veins
- Pediatric patients
- Elderly patients
- Lower needle insertion angle

✋ **ALERT:** Observe your facility's policy for routine use of winged blood collection sets.

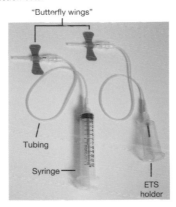

"Butterfly wings"

Tubing

Syringe

ETS holder

Additional Equipment

- Tourniquets
- Gloves
- Antiseptics
  - 70% isopropyl alcohol (for routine blood collection)
  - Chlorhexidine gluconate or iodine (for procedures requiring additional sterility, such as blood cultures)

- 2-inch × 2-inch gauze
- Bandages
- Pen
- Slides
- Biohazard transport bags
- Hand sanitizers

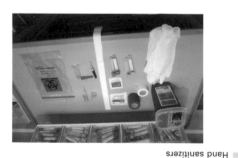

Equipment Quality Control

- Visually inspect each needle for:
  - Sealed sterile package
  - Nonpointed or barbed needles
- Check tubes' expiration dates because use of expired tubes can cause:
  - Incompletely filled tubes, resulting in:
    - Dilution of specimen by liquid anticoagulant
    - Distortion of cellular structures by increased chemical concentrations
  - Clotted anticoagulated specimens
  - Improperly preserved specimens
  - Insecure gel barriers

Equipment Notes

Workplace 1 Policies

_____

_____

_____

_____

_____

_____

_____

_____

Workplace 2 Policies

_____

_____

_____

_____

_____

_____

_____

_____

VENIPUNCTURE CHECKLIST

- Obtain and examine the requisition form.
- Greet the patient, and state the procedure to be done.
- Identify the patient using two identifiers.
- Select the correct tubes and puncturing equipment for the procedure.
- Sanitize hands.
- Apply gloves.
- Position the patient's arm, and apply the tourniquet.
- Ask the patient to make a fist, and select the venipuncture site by palpation.
- Release the tourniquet.
- Cleanse the site.
- Assemble the equipment.
- Reapply the tourniquet.
- Remove the needle cap and examine the needle.
- Anchor the vein below the puncture site.
- Insert the needle with the bevel up.
- Push the evacuated tube completely into the holder.
- Collect the specimens in the **correct order of draw**.
- Gently invert the specimens three to eight times immediately after collection.
- Ask the patient to release the fist.
- Release the tourniquet within 1 minute.
- Place gauze over the needle, remove the needle, and apply pressure.
- Activate the needle safety device.
- Dispose of the needle in the sharps disposal container.
- Label the tubes, and confirm with the patient or ID band.
- Examine the patient's puncture site and apply a bandage.
- Prepare the specimens and requisition forms for transportation to the laboratory, making sure to observe special handling instructions.
- Dispose of used supplies.
- Remove gloves.
- Sanitize hands.
- Thank the patient.

Common Venipuncture Veins

Arm Veins

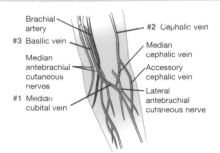

Brachial artery

#3 Basilic vein

Median antebrachial cutaneous nerves

#1 Median cubital vein

#2 Cephalic vein

Median cephalic vein

Accessory cephalic vein

Lateral antebrachial cutaneous nerve

Hand Veins

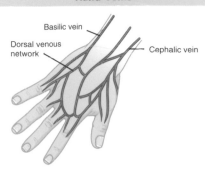

Basilic vein

Dorsal venous network

Cephalic vein

AREAS TO AVOID

Certain areas must be avoided for venipuncture because of the possibility of decreased blood flow, infection, hemolysis, specimen contamination, or injury to the patient. These areas include:

- Underside of the wrist
- Occluded veins
- Edematous areas
- Hematomas
- Burned or scarred areas
- Arm located on the same side as a recent mastectomy
- Arm that contains an IV
- Arm that contains cannulas or fistulas
- Foot or leg veins (without documented permission of the physician)

✋ **ALERT:** Leg and foot veins are more susceptible to infection and thrombi formation in patients with diabetes, cardiac problems, and coagulation disorders.

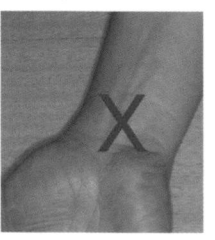 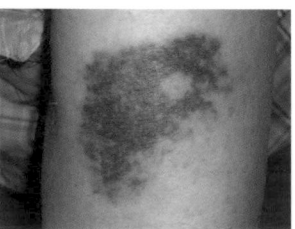

METHODS OF VEIN ENHANCEMENT

- Massage the arm upward from the wrist to the elbows.
- Briefly hang the arm down.
- Apply heat to the site for 3 to 5 minutes.

Patient Identification

ALERT: The Clinical and Laboratory Standards Institute (CLSI), College of American Pathologists (CAP), and The Joint Commission (TJC) recommend two patient identifiers when collecting blood.

For a Hospitalized Patient

1. Verbally identify the patient by asking the patient to state his or her full name, spell the last name, and state their birthdate.
2. Check that the information on the patient's ID band matches the information on the requisition form, including:
   - Patient's name
   - Hospital identification number
   - Date of birth
   - Physician

ALERT: Verify any discrepancies between the patient's ID band and the requisition form *before* performing venipuncture.

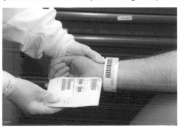

For an Outpatient

- Verbally identify the patient by asking the patient to state his or her full name; spell the last name; or give address, birth date, or unique identification number.
- Compare the response to the requisition form.
- Check the patient's photo identification, if required.
- Check the patient's ID band or patient ID card, if available.

👋 ALERT: Verify any discrepancies between the patient's ID and the requisition form *before* performing venipuncture.

Patient Positioning

■ Ask the patient to sit or lie down.

👋 ALERT: Never draw blood from a patient who is standing.

When Using an Arm Vein
■ Position the patient's arm so that it is firmly supported and slightly bent in a downward position. This positioning allows the tubes to fill from the bottom up, preventing reflux and additive carryover between tubes.

👋 ALERT: Make sure that the patient does not hyperextend the arm.

SUPPORTING THE ARM WITH A FIST

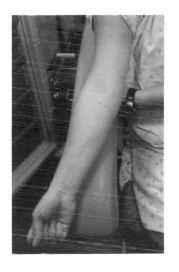

SUPPORTING THE ARM WITH A WEDGE

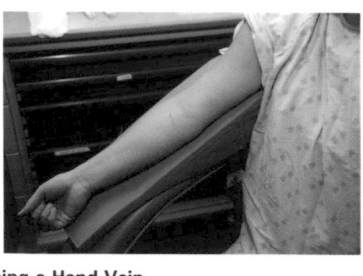

When Using a Hand Vein
- Support the hand on the bed or drawing chair armrest.
- Ask the patient to make a loose fist.

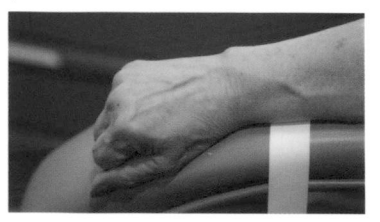

Tourniquet Application

Equipment

- Non-latex tourniquet

ALERT: Always check for possible latex allergies before applying a latex tourniquet, if a non-latex tourniquet is unavailable.

✋ **ALERT:** When using a blood pressure cuff as a tourniquet, inflate it to just below the diastolic blood pressure.

Procedure

1. Position the tourniquet 3 to 4 inches above the venipuncture site.

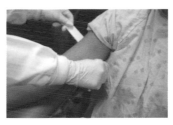

2. Grasp both sides of the tourniquet and, while maintaining tension, cross the tourniquet over the patient's arm.

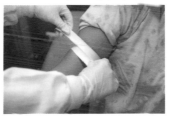

33

3. Hold both ends of the tourniquet between the thumb and forefinger of one hand close to the arm.

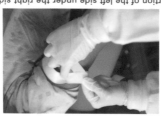

4. Tuck a portion of the left side under the right side to make a partial loop facing the antecubital area.

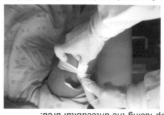

5. Verify that the tourniquet is properly applied by checking that the ends point up and away from the venipuncture site.

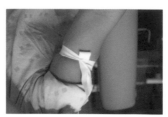

✋ **ALERT**: Do not leave a tourniquet in place for longer than 1 minute because hemoconcentration and hemolysis can occur.

Palpating the Vein

- Use the tip of the index finger of the nondominant hand.
- Use a pushing motion, rather than a stroking motion.
- Feel the vein in both a vertical and horizontal direction.

✋ **ALERT**: Never use the thumb for palpation because it has a pulse.

PALPATING AN ARM VEIN

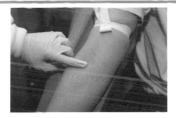

PALPATING A HAND VEIN

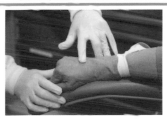

Anchoring the Vein

- Anchoring the vein keeps the skin taut and prevents the vein from slipping ("rolling") when the needle is inserted.

Arm Vein

- Place the thumb of your nondominant hand 1 to 2 inches below and slightly to the side of the insertion site.
- Place your four fingers on the back of the patient's arm.

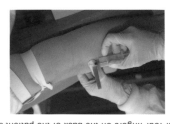

Hand Vein

- Ask the patient to make a fist or to grab the end of the drawing chair arm.
- Pull the skin tightly over the knuckles with the thumb of your nondominant hand.

Venipuncture Using an ETS

Equipment

- Requisition form
- Gloves
- Evacuated tube needle with safety device
- Evacuated tube holder
- Tourniquet
- 70% isopropyl alcohol pads
- Evacuated tube needle (with safety device if the needle does not have one)

■ Evacuated tubes
■ 2-inch × 2-inch gauze
■ Sharps disposal container
■ Indelible pen
■ Bandage
■ Biohazard transport bag

Procedure

1. Obtain and examine the requisition form. Check for completeness, date and time of collection, and priority.

👋 **ALERT:** Never collect a specimen without a requisition form.

2. Greet the patient, explain the procedure, and obtain patient's consent.
3. Identify the patient verbally by having him or her state both the first and last names, spell the last name, and give the date of birth. Compare the information on the patient's ID band with the information on the requisition form. A minimum of two identifiers is required.

👋 **ALERT:** Verify discrepancies between the patient's ID band and the requisition form *before* drawing blood.

4. Verify the patient's adherence to pretest preparation, such as dietary and medication restrictions. Ask about latex allergies.

👋 **ALERT:** Report irregularities according to your facility's protocol before collecting the specimen.

5. Confirm that the patient has removed all objects from his or her mouth.
6. Select the correct tubes and other equipment for the procedure, making sure to keep extra tubes available. Place on your non-dominant side.
7. Sanitize your hands using the proper technique.
8. Apply gloves.
9. Position the patient's arm or hand in preparation for venipuncture.

👋 **ALERT:** Make sure that the patient does not hyperextend the arm.

10. Ask the patient to make a fist.
11. Apply a tourniquet 3 to 4 inches above the venipuncture site.
12. Palpate the area with the index finger of the nondominant hand in a vertical and horizontal direction to locate a large vein and to determine the depth, direction, and size.
   - The median cubital vein is the first choice, followed by the cephalic vein.
   - The basilic vein should be avoided if possible.
13. Remove the tourniquet.
   👆 ALERT: Do not leave the tourniquet in place for longer than 1 minute to prevent hemoconcentration and hemolysis.
14. Ask the patient to open the fist to prevent hemoconcentration.
15. Cleanse the site with 70% isopropyl alcohol in a back and forth motion, moving outward 2 to 2 in., creating a friction and allow the site to air-dry for maximum bacteriostatic action.
   👆 ALERT: Position all supplies within easy reach on your non-dominant side to avoid reaching over venipuncture site. Reaching over to retrieve supplies may cause painful or damaging needle movement.
16. Assemble the equipment while the alcohol is drying:
   ■ Attach the multisample needle to the holder.

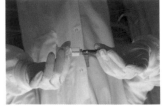

   ■ Insert the tube into the holder up to the tube advancement mark or wait until after needle entry into the vein.

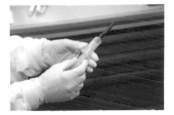

17. Reapply the tourniquet.

👋 **ALERT:** Do not touch the puncture site with an unclean finger. Clean the gloved finger in the same manner as the venipuncture site, if necessary.

18. Ask the patient to remake a fist, but instruct the patient not to "pump" or "continuously clench" the fist to prevent hemoconcentration.

19. Remove the plastic needle cap and examine the needle for defects, such as nonpointed or barbed ends. Discard the needle if it is flawed.

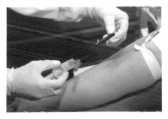

20. Anchor the vein by placing the thumb of your nondominant hand 1 to 2 inches below the site and pulling the skin taut.
21. Grasp the assembled needle and tube holder using your dominant hand, with the thumb on the top near the hub and your other fingers beneath.

👋 **ALERT**: Brace your fingers against the patient's arm to prevent movement of the needle when changing tubes.

22. Smoothly insert the needle into the vein at a 15- to 30-degree angle with the bevel up until you feel a lessening of resistance.

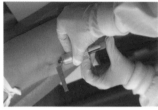

23. Using your thumb, advance the tube onto the back of the evacuated tube needle while your index and middle fingers grasp the flared ends of the holder.

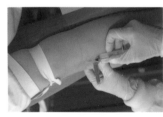

24. When blood flows into the tube, release the tourniquet and ask the patient to open the fist.

25. Gently remove the tube when the blood stops flowing into it.

👋 **ALERT**: Fill each tube to the correct fill line.

🖐 **ALERT**: Gently invert anticoagulated tubes three to eight times as soon as they are removed from the holder.

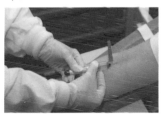

26. Insert the next tube using the **correct order of draw**.
27. Remove the last tube collected from the holder before removing the needle from the vein and then gently invert the tube.
28. Cover the puncture site with clean gauze.
29. Remove the needle smoothly and apply pressure or ask the patient to apply pressure if capable.

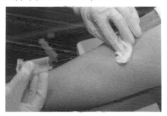

30. After removing the needle from the vein, immediately activate the safety device following the manufacturer's guidelines.

👈 **ALERT:** Do not recap, cut, or bend needles.

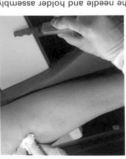

31. Dispose of the needle and holder assembly into a sharps disposal container.

👈 **ALERT:** Do not separate the needle from the blood tube holder.

32. Before leaving an inpatient's room, label the tubes and reconfirm the patient's identification.

👈 **ALERT:** Do not release outpatients before labeling the tubes and confirming the labeled tubes with the patient's identification.

33. Examine the puncture site to verify that the bleeding has stopped.

👈 **ALERT:** Watch for hematoma formation by visually observing for subcutaneous bleeding *before* applying a bandage. Hematoma formation can place pressure on the nerves and cause a disabling compression nerve injury.

34. Apply a bandage. Place a bandage over folded gauze for additional pressure.

35. Prepare the specimens and requisition forms for transportation to the laboratory, making sure to follow special handling instructions.

36. Dispose of used supplies.
37. Thank the patient.
38. Remove your gloves.
39. Sanitize your hands.

Evacuated Tube System Collection Notes

_____

_____

_____

_____

_____

_____

_____

_____

_____

_____

_____

_____

_____

_____

_____

_____

_____

_____

Venipuncture Using a Syringe

Equipment

- Requisition form
- Gloves
- Tourniquet
- 70% isopropyl alcohol pad
- Syringe needle with safety device
- Syringe
- Blood transfer device
- Evacuated tubes
- 2-inch × 2-inch gauze
- Sharps disposal container
- Indelible pen
- Bandage
- Biohazard transport bag

Procedure

1. Obtain and examine the requisition form. Check for completeness, date and time of collection, and priority.

✋ ALERT: Never collect a specimen without a requisition form.

2. Greet the patient, explain the procedure, and obtain patient's consent.
3. Identify the patient verbally by having him or her state both the first and last names, spell the last name, and give the date of birth. Compare the information on the patient's ID band with the information on the requisition form. A minimum of two identifiers is required.

✋ ALERT: Verify discrepancies between the patient's ID band and the requisition form *before* drawing blood.

4. Verify the patient's adherence to pretest preparation, such as dietary and medication restrictions. Ask about latex allergies.

✋ ALERT: Report irregularities according to your facility's protocol before collecting the specimens.

5. Confirm that the patient has removed all objects from his or her mouth.
6. Select the correct tubes and other equipment for the procedure, making sure to keep extra tubes available.
7. Sanitize your hands using the proper technique.

8. Apply gloves.
9. Position the patient's arm or hand in preparation for venipuncture.

ALERT: Make sure that the patient does not hyperextend the arm.

10. Ask the patient to make a fist.
11. Apply a tourniquet 3 to 4 inches above the venipuncture site.
12. Palpate the area with the index finger of the nondominant hand in a vertical and horizontal direction to locate a large vein and to determine the depth, direction, and size.
    - The median cubital vein is the first choice, followed by the cephalic vein.
    - The basilic vein should be avoided if possible.
13. Remove the tourniquet.

ALERT: Do not leave the tourniquet in place for longer than 1 minute to prevent hemoconcentration and hemolysis.

14. Ask the patient to open his or her fist to prevent hemoconcentration.
15. Cleanse the site with 70% isopropyl alcohol in a back and forth motion, moving outward 2 to 3 in., creating a friction, and allow the site to air-dry for maximum bacteriostatic action.
16. Assemble the equipment as the alcohol is drying:
    - Select the syringe size according to the volume of blood required for testing.
    - Attach the hypodermic needle to the syringe.
    - Pull the plunger back to ensure that it moves freely and then push it forward to remove any air in the syringe.

ALERT: Position all supplies within easy reach on your non-dominant side to avoid reaching over venipuncture site. Reaching over to retrieve supplies may cause painful or damaging needle movement.

17. Reapply the tourniquet.
18. Remove the needle cap and inspect the needle.
19. Ask the patient to remake a fist, but instruct the patient not to "pump" or "continuously clench" the fist to prevent hemoconcentration.

🔔 **ALERT:** Do not touch the puncture site with an unclean finger. Clean the gloved finger in the same manner as the venipuncture site, if necessary.

20. Anchor the vein by placing the thumb of your nondominant hand 1 to 2 inches below the site and pulling the skin taut.

21. Hold the syringe in your dominant hand with your thumb on top near the hub and the other fingers underneath, as you would an ETS holder.

22. Smoothly insert the needle into the vein at a 15- to 30-degree angle with the bevel up until you feel a lessening of resistance. A flash of blood will appear in the syringe hub when the vein has been entered.

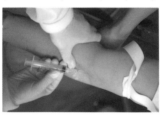

23. Pull back the syringe plunger using your nondominant hand to collect the appropriate amount of blood.

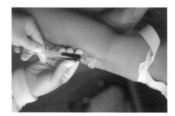

24. Brace your fingers against the patient's arm to prevent movement of the needle when pulling back on the plunger of the syringe.

👋 **ALERT:** Pulling the plunger of the syringe back too slowly can cause the blood to begin to clot before the collection is completed.

👋 **ALERT:** Pulling the plunger of the syringe back too quickly can cause hemolysis or a vein to collapse.

25. Release the tourniquet and ask the patient to open the fist.
26. Cover the puncture site with gauze.
27. Remove the needle smoothly, and immediately activate the safety device following the manufacturer's guidelines.

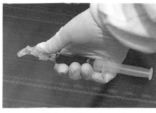

28. Apply pressure or ask the patient to apply pressure if capable.
29. Remove the needle from the syringe and discard it in a sharps disposal container.
30. Attach a blood transfer device to the syringe.

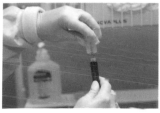

🖐 **ALERT:** Do not recap, cut, or bend needles.

🖐 **ALERT:** Quickly transfer the blood from the syringe to the evacuated tube to prevent clotting.

31. Holding the syringe vertically with the blood transfer device at the bottom, advance the evacuated tube onto the internal needle in the blood transfer device.

🖐 **ALERT:** Keep the tube in a vertical position to ensure that the tubes fill from the bottom up to avoid cross-contamination.

🖐 **ALERT:** Do not push on the plunger.

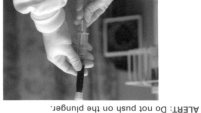

32. Fill tubes in the same order as the ETS system.
33. Mix anticoagulated tubes by gentle inversion three to eight times as soon as they are filled.
34. After the tubes are filled, discard the entire syringe and blood transfer device into a sharps disposal container.
35. Before leaving the patient, label the tubes and reconfirm the patient's identification.

🖐 **ALERT:** Do not release outpatients before labeling the tubes and confirming the labeled tubes with the patient's identification.

36. Examine the puncture site to verify that the bleeding has stopped.

🖐 **ALERT:** Watch for hematoma formation by visually observing for subcutaneous bleeding *before* applying a bandage. Hematoma formation can place pressure on the nerves and cause a disabling compression nerve injury.

37. Apply a bandage. Place a bandage over folded gauze for additional pressure.
38. Prepare the specimens and requisition forms for transportation to the laboratory, making sure to observe special handling instructions.
39. Dispose of used supplies.
40. Thank the patient.
41. Remove your gloves.
42. Sanitize your hands.

Syringe Collection Notes

_____

_____

_____

_____

_____

_____

_____

_____

_____

_____

_____

_____

_____

_____

Venipuncture Using a Winged Blood Collection Set

Equipment

- Requisition form
- Gloves
- Tourniquet
- 70% isopropyl alcohol pad
- Winged blood collection set
- Syringe or evacuated tube holder
- Blood transfer device
- Evacuated tubes
- 2-inch × 2-inch gauze
- Sharps disposal container
- Indelible pen
- Bandage
- Biohazard transport bag

Procedure

1. Obtain and examine the requisition form. Check for completeness, date and time of collection, and priority.

👋 **ALERT:** Never collect a specimen without a requisition form.

2. Greet the patient, explain the procedure, and obtain patient's consent.

3. Identify the patient verbally by having him or her state both the first and last names, spell the last name, and give the date of birth. Compare the information on the patient's ID band with the information on the requisition form. A minimum of two identifiers is required.

👋 **ALERT:** Verify discrepancies between the patient's ID band and the requisition form *before drawing blood*.

4. Verify the patient's adherence to pretest preparation, such as dietary and medication restrictions. Ask about latex allergies.

👋 **ALERT:** Report irregularities according to your facility's protocol before collecting the specimen.

5. Confirm that the patient has removed all objects from his or her mouth.

6. Select the correct tubes and other equipment for the procedure, making sure to keep extra tubes available.

7. Sanitize your hands using the proper technique.
8. Apply gloves.
9. Position the patient's arm or hand in preparation for venipuncture.

✋ ALERT: Make sure that the patient does not hyperextend the arm.

10. Ask the patient to make a fist.
11. Apply a tourniquet 3 to 4 inches above the venipuncture site.
12. Palpate the area with the index finger of the nondominant hand in a vertical and horizontal direction to locate a large vein and to determine the depth, direction, and size.
    ■ The median cubital vein is the first choice, followed by the cephalic vein.
    ■ The basilic vein should be avoided if possible.
13. Remove the tourniquet.

✋ ALERT: Do not leave the tourniquet in place for longer than 1 minute to prevent hemoconcentration and hemolysis.

14. Ask the patient to open his or her fist to prevent hemoconcentration.
15. Cleanse the site with 70% isopropyl alcohol in a back and forth motion, moving outward 2 to 3 in. creating a friction, and allow the site to air-dry for maximum bacteriostatic action.
16. Assemble the equipment while the alcohol is drying:
    ■ Attach the winged blood collection set to an evacuated tube holder *or* syringe.
    ■ Stretch out the coiled plastic tubing.
    ■ If using a syringe, pull the plunger back to ensure that it moves freely and then push it forward to remove any air in the syringe.

✋ ALERT: Position all supplies within easy reach on your nondominant side to avoid reaching over venipuncture site. Reaching over to retrieve supplies may cause painful or damaging needle movement.

    ■ If using an evacuated tube holder, insert the first tube to the tube advancement mark.

🖐 **ALERT:** To avoid an accidental needlestick, be sure to attach the evacuated tube holder and not just push the tubes onto the back of the rubber-sheathed needle.

17. Reapply the tourniquet.

18. Ask the patient to remake a fist, but instruct the patient not to "pump," or "continuously clinch" the fist to prevent hemoconcentration.

19. Remove the needle cap and inspect the needle.

20. Lay the syringe or evacuated tube holder and tubing next to the patient's hand.

🖐 **ALERT:** Do not touch the puncture site with an unclean finger. Clean the gloved finger in the same manner as the venipuncture site, if necessary.

21. Anchor the vein.

22. Grasp the needle between your thumb and index finger by holding the back of the needle or by folding the wings together.

23. Smoothly insert the needle into the vein at a shallow 10- to 15-degree angle with the bevel up.

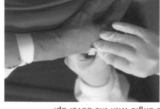

24. Thread the needle into the lumen of the vein until the bevel is firmly "seated" in the vein. Watch for a flash of blood, which appears in the tubing when the needle has entered the vein.

25. When using a syringe, pull back on the plunger of the syringe slowly and smoothly with your nondominant hand to collect the blood.

🖐 **ALERT:** Do not pull back on the syringe plunger if a blood flash does not appear.

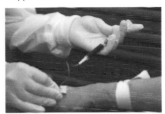

26. When using an evacuated tube holder, insert the tubes onto the back of the needle in the holder in the **correct order of draw**.

🖐 **ALERT:** Always use a discard tube when collecting light blue tubes. Doing so primes the tubing to maintain the correct blood-to-anticoagulant ratio.

🖐 **ALERT:** Gently invert anticoagulated tubes three to eight times as soon as they are removed from the holder.

27. Release the tourniquet and ask the patient to open the fist.
28. Cover the puncture site with clean gauze.
29. Remove the needle smoothly.

🖐 **ALERT:** When removing a winged blood collection needle from a vein, always hold the base of the needle or the wings until you dispose of the set in a sharps disposal container.

30. Activate the needle safety device following the manufacturer's guidelines.

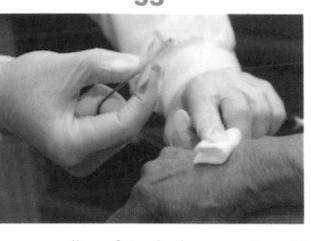

👆 **ALERT**: Some needle safety devices can be activated before the needle is removed from the vein.

👆 **ALERT**: Do not recap, cut, or bend needles.

31. Apply pressure or ask the patient to apply pressure to the site.
32. When using a syringe, remove the winged blood collection set from the syringe and discard it in a sharps disposal container.
33. Attach a blood transfer device to the syringe.

👆 **ALERT**: Quickly transfer the blood from the syringe to the evacuated tube to prevent clotting.

34. Holding the syringe vertically with the blood transfer device at the bottom, advance the evacuated tube onto the internal needle in the blood transfer device.

ALERT: Keep the tube in a vertical position to ensure that the tubes fill from the bottom up to avoid cross-contamination.

ALERT: Do not push on the plunger.

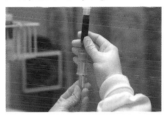

35. Fill the evacuated tubes in the **correct order of draw**.

ALERT: Gently invert anticoagulated tubes three to eight times as soon as they are removed from the transfer device.

36. After filling the tubes, discard the syringe and blood transfer device in a sharps disposal container.
37. Before leaving the patient, label the tubes and reconfirm the patient's identification.

ALERT· Do not release outpatients before labeling the tubes and confirming the labeled tubes with the patient's identification.

38. Examine the puncture site to verify that the bleeding has stopped.

ALERT: Watch for hematoma formation by visually observing for subcutaneous bleeding *before* applying a bandage. Hematoma formation can place pressure on the nerves and cause a disabling compression nerve injury.

39. Apply a bandage. Place a bandage over folded gauze for additional pressure.
40. Prepare the specimens and requisition forms for transportation to the laboratory, making sure to observe special handling instructions.

41. Dispose of used supplies.
42. Thank the patient.
43. Remove your gloves.
44. Sanitize your hands.

Winged Blood Collection Notes

_____

_____

_____

_____

_____

_____

_____

_____

_____

_____

_____

_____

_____

_____

_____

_____

_____

_____

Major Tests Affected by Patient Pre-examination Variables

Variable	Increased Results	Decreased Results
Age	• Cholesterol • Triglycerides	• Hormones
Alcohol	• Alanine transaminase (ALT) • Aldosterone • Aspartate aminotransferase (AST) • Catecholamine • Cholesterol • Cortisol • Estradiol • Glucose • High-density lipoprotein (HDL) • Iron • Luteinizing hormone (LH) • Mean corpuscular volume (MCV) • Prolactin • Triglycerides	• Testosterone
Altitude	• Hematocrit • Hemoglobin • Red blood cells (RBCs)	
Caffeine	• Fatty acids • Glycerol • Hormone levels • Lipoproteins • Serum gastrin	

Continued

Variable	Increased Results	Decreased Results
Dehydration	• Calcium • Coagulation factors • Enzymes • Iron • Red blood cells • Sodium	
Diurnal variation (a.m.)	• Aldosterone • Bilirubin • Cortisol • Estradiol • Follicle-stimulating hormone (FSH) • Hemoglobin • Insulin • LH • Potassium • RBCs • Renin • Serum iron • Testosterone • Thyroid-stimulating hormone (TSH)	• Creatinine • Eosinophils • Glucose • Phosphate • Triglycerides
Exercise, long-term	• Aldolase • AST • Creatine kinase (CK) • Creatinine • Lactate dehydrogenase (LD) • Sex hormones	

Continued

Variable	Increased Results	Decreased Results
Exercise, short-term	• Aldosterone • Angiotensin • AST • Bilirubin • CK • Creatinine • Fatty acids • HDL • Hormones • Insulin • Lactic acid • LD • Potassium • Renin • Uric acid • WBCs	• Arterial pH • Partial pressure of carbon dioxide (P_{CO_2})
Nonfasting	• AST • Bilirubin • Blood urea nitrogen (BUN) • Cholesterol • Glucose • Growth hormone (GH) • HDL • Low-density lipoprotein (LDL) • Phosphorus • Triglycerides • Uric acid	
Prolonged fasting	• Bilirubin • Fatty acids • Glucagon • Ketones • Lactate • Triglycerides	• Cholesterol • Glucose • Insulin • Thyroid hormones

Continued

Variable	Increased Results	Decreased Results
Posture	• Albumin • Aldosterone • Bilirubin • Calcium • Catecholamines • Cholesterol • Cortisol • Enzymes • Iron thyroxine (T_4), plasma renin • RBCs • Serum aldosterone • Total protein • Triglycerides • White blood cells (WBCs)	
Pregnancy	• Erythrocyte sedimentation rate (ESR) • Factors II, V, VII, IX, and X	• Protein • Alkaline phosphatase (ALP) • Estradiol • Free fatty acids • RBCs • Iron
Smoking	• ALP • BUN • Catecholamines • Cholesterol • Cortisol • GH • Glucose • Hematocrit • Hemoglobin • Immunoglobulin (Ig) E	• Ig A • Ig G • Ig M

Continued

Variable	Increased Results	Decreased Results
	• RBCs • Triglycerides • WBCs	
Stress	• Adrenal hormones • Aldosterone • GH • Partial pressure of oxygen (Po_2) • Prolactin • Renin • TSH • WBCs	• Partial pressure of carbon dioxide (Pco_2) • Serum iron

Effects of Medications on Laboratory Tests

Medications	Affected Tests Results
Acetaminophen and certain antibiotics	• Elevated liver enzymes and bilirubin levels
Aspirin, salicylates, and herbal supplements	• Prolonged PT and bleeding time
Certain antibiotics	• Elevated BUN and creatinine levels and electrolyte imbalance
Chemotherapy	• Decreased RBCs, WBCs, and platelet levels
Cholesterol-lowering drugs	• Prolonged PT and APTT

Continued

COMPLI-
CATIONS

Medications	Affected Tests Results
Corticosteroids and estrogen diuretics	• Elevated amylase and lipase levels
Diuretics	• Increased calcium, glucose, and uric acid levels and decreased sodium and potassium levels
Fluorescein dye	• Increased creatinine, cortisol, and digoxin levels
Opiates	• Increased liver and pancreatic enzyme levels
Oral contraceptives	• Decreased apoprotein, transcortin, cholesterol, HDL, triglyceride, LH, FSH, ferritin, vitamin B_{12}, and iron levels • Elevated erythrocyte sedimentation rate (ESR)

HERBS, VITAMINS, AND DIETARY SUPPLEMENTS THAT AFFECT COAGULATION AND CLOTTING

- Alfalfa
- Anise
- Bilberry
- Bladder wrack
- Bromelain
- Cat's claw
- Celery
- Coenzyme Q10
- Coleus
- Cordyceps
- Danshen
- Dong quai
- Evening primrose
- Fenugreek
- Feverfew
- *Fucus*
- Garlic
- Ginger
- Ginkgo biloba

- Ginseng
- Grape seed
- Green tea
- Guarana
- Horse chestnut seed
- Horseradish
- Horsetail rush
- Licorice
- Omega-3 fatty acids in fish oil
- Prickly ash
- Red clover
- Reishi mushroom
- St. John's wort
- Sweet clover
- Turmeric
- Vitamin E
- White willow

ALERT: Be sure to ask the patient about the use of these over-the-counter products, especially when excessive postvenipuncture bleeding occurs.

Failure to Obtain Blood

Cause	Remedy
Bevel against the upper wall of the vein	Remove the evacuated tube and rotate the needle a quarter of a turn.
Bevel against the lower wall of the vein	Remove the evacuated tube and rotate the needle a quarter of a turn.

Skin   Vein

Skin   Vein

Continued

Failure to Obtain Blood—cont'd

Cause	Remedy
Needle inserted too far (too deep) 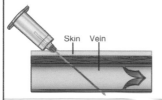	Gently pull the needle back.
Needle partially inserted (too shallow) 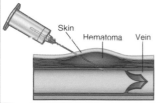	Slowly advance the needle into the vein.
Collapsed vein 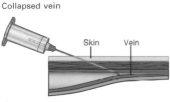	Use a smaller evacuated tube, a syringe, or a winged blood collection set.

Continued

Failure to Obtain Blood—cont'd

Cause	Remedy
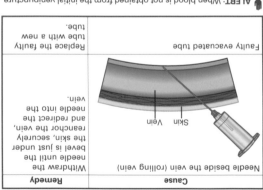 Needle beside the vein (rolling vein)	Withdraw the needle until the bevel is just under the skin, securely reanchor the vein, and redirect the needle into the vein.
Faulty evacuated tube	Replace the faulty tube with a new tube.

🖐 **ALERT:** When blood is not obtained from the initial venipuncture, the blood collector should select another site and repeat the procedure using a new needle.

🖐 **ALERT:** According to the Clinical and Laboratory Standards Institute (CLSI) standard (GP41), another person should be asked to collect the specimens if a successful collection is not obtained after two attempts.

Patient Complications

Fainting (Syncope)

Signs and Symptoms

- Nausea
- Paleness of the skin
- Hyperventilation
- Light-headedness
- Dizziness
- Feeling of warmth
- Cold, clammy skin

Recommended Actions
- Immediately remove the tourniquet and needle.
- Apply pressure to the site.
- Lower the patient's head.
- Keep the patient in the area for 15 to 30 minutes.
- Document the incident

✋ **ALERT:** Ask a patient with a history of fainting to lie down during blood collection.

✋ **ALERT:** According to the CLSI standards (GP41), the use of ammonia inhalants may be associated with adverse effects and is not recommended.

Patient Refusal

Recommended Actions
- Be aware that the patient has the legal right to refuse venipuncture and may do so for religious or cultural beliefs.
- Watch for nonverbal body language that may indicate patient refusal.
- Stress the importance of the laboratory test to the patient.
- Document the refusal on the requisition form.
- Notify the nursing staff.

Petechiae

Signs and Symptoms
- Small, nonraised red spots
  - Appear when tourniquet is applied
  - May indicate a vascular or platelet disorder

Recommended Actions
- Apply additional pressure after needle removal.

✋ **ALERT:** Be aware that the presence of petechiae may indicate prolonged bleeding following venipuncture.

Seizures

Signs and Symptoms
- Sudden uncontrollable movements
- Convulsions

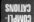
Technical Errors Affecting the Patient

Infection

Causes

- Failure to use aseptic technique
- Site contact with nonsterile finger or gauze

Recommended Actions

- Instruct the patient to keep the bandage on for at least 15 minutes after venipuncture.
- Do not open bandages ahead of time or place them on a table or lab coat.
- Clean the palpating finger in the same manner as the site was cleaned if additional palpation is required.
- Perform the venipuncture immediately after removing the needle cap.

Nerve Injury

Temporary or permanent nerve damage can be caused by errors in technique and may result in loss of movement in the arm or hand.

Symptoms

- Shooting pain
- Electric-like tingling
- Numbness of the arm
- Pain that radiates up or down the arm

Recommended Actions

- Remove the tourniquet and needle.
- Apply pressure to the site.
- Summon help.
- Restrain the patient only to the extent needed to prevent injury.
- Do not place anything in the patient's mouth.
- Document the time the seizure started and stopped.

Causes

- Blind probing for the vein
- Selection of high-risk venipuncture sites (e.g., underside of the wrist, basilic vein)
- Insertion of the needle at an angle greater than 30 degrees
- Lateral redirection of the needle
- Jerky movements of the needle
- Movement by the patient while the needle is in the vein
- Pressure from a hematoma
- Tourniquet that is on too long or is too tight

Recommended Actions

- Follow CLSI standards for site selection.
- Immediately discontinue the venipuncture.
- Apply a cold ice pack after needle removal.
- Document the incident.
- Follow facility policy.

Hematomas

Hematomas are caused by errors in technique that lead to the leakage of blood into the tissues around the venipuncture site.

Causes

- Failure to remove the tourniquet prior to removing the needle
- Application of inadequate pressure to the site after needle removal
- Bending the patient's arm while applying pressure
- Excessive probing to locate the vein
- Failure to insert the needle far enough into the vein
- Insertion of the needle through the vein
- Use of a needle too large for the vein
- Use of veins that are small and fragile
- Accidental puncture of the brachial artery

Recommended Actions

- Discontinue the venipuncture immediately.
- Apply pressure to the site for 2 minutes.
- Offer a cold compress to minimize swelling and pain.
- Follow facility policy.

69

Compartment Syndrome

Compartment syndrome is caused by blood accumulating within the tissues of the muscles that surround the arm or hand, resulting in a buildup of pressure that interferes with blood flow and causes muscle or nerve injury.

Symptoms

- Pain
- Swelling
- Numbness
- Permanent nerve injury

Causes

- Excessive bleeding in a patient receiving an anticoagulant
- Excessive bleeding in a patient with a coagulation disorder
- Failure to check for bleeding or hematoma formation before applying a bandage

Recommended Actions

- Before performing venipuncture, ask the patient whether he or she is receiving anticoagulant therapy.
- Maintain pressure on the site until bleeding has stopped.

Accidental Arterial Puncture

Signs

- Appearance of bright-red blood spurting into the tube
- Hematoma formation

Causes

- Probing to find the vein
- Lateral movement of the needle near the basilic vein

Recommended Actions

- Discontinue the venipuncture.
- Apply pressure to the site for 5 minutes (possibly 10 minutes if the patient is on anticoagulant therapy) or until bleeding stops.
- ALERT: Note on the requisition form that the specimen may be arterial blood because some test values are different for arterial blood.

Technical Errors Affecting the Specimen

Technical complications with the venipuncture procedure can result in inaccurate test results, an inability to obtain blood, discomfort to the patient, and a rejected specimen.

Hemoconcentration

In hemoconcentration, the plasma portion of the blood passes into the tissue, which increases the concentration of protein-analytes in the peripheral blood affecting test results.

Causes

- Prolonged tourniquet application (longer than 1 minute)
- Site probing
- Long-term IV therapy
- Occluded veins
- Vigorous fist pumping

Increased Test Results

- Ammonia
- Bilirubin
- Calcium
- Enzymes
- Iron
- Lactic acid
- Lipids
- Potassium
- Proteins
- Red blood cells

🖐 **ALERT:** Because lactic acid tests are extremely sensitive to venous stasis, tourniquet application and fist clenching are not recommended when drawing specimens for these tests.

Laboratory Tests Affected by Hemolysis

Seriously Affected	Noticeably Affected	Slightly Affected
Aspartate aminotransferase (AST)	Activated partial thromboplastin time (APTT)	Albumin Alkaline phosphatase
Complete blood count (CBC)	Alanine aminotransferase (ALT)	Bilirubin Calcium (Ca)
Lactic dehydrogenase (LD)	C-peptide	Haptoglobin Magnesium (Mg)
Potassium (K)	Creatine kinase (CK)	Phosphorus (P)
Troponin (T)	Serum iron (FE)	Rapid plasma reagin (RPR)
	Prothrombin time (PT) Thyroxine (T₄)	Total protein (TP)

✋ **ALERT:** Hemolysis can be detected by the presence of pink or red plasma or serum.

✋ **ALERT:** Even hemolysis that is not evident to the naked eye can elevate critical potassium values.

Causes

Errors in Performance

■ Use of a needle with a too-small diameter (above 23 gauge)
■ Use of a small needle with a large evacuated tube
■ Use of an improperly attached needle on a syringe so that frothing occurs as the blood enters the syringe
■ Pulling back of the syringe plunger too fast
■ Drawing of blood from a site containing a hematoma
■ Vigorous mixing of tubes
■ Forcing of blood from a syringe into an evacuated tube
■ Collection of specimens from an IV line when not recommended by the manufacturer
■ Application of the tourniquet too close to the puncture site or for too long a time

- Use of fragile hand veins
- Performance of venipuncture before alcohol dries
- Collection of blood through different internal diameters of catheter and connectors
- Partial filling of sodium fluoride tubes
- Readjustment of the needle in the vein (vigorous probing)
- Use of occluded veins

Problems With Processing, Handling, or Transporting the Specimen
- Rimming of a clotted specimen
- Prolonged contact of serum or plasma with cells
- Centrifugation at a higher-than-recommended speed and with increased heat exposure in the centrifuge
- Elevated or decreased blood temperatures
- Use of pneumatic tube systems with unpadded canisters, speed acceleration or deceleration, or excessive agitation

Patient Physiological Factors
- Metabolic disorders
  - Liver disease
  - Sickle cell anemia
  - Autoimmune hemolytic anemia
  - Blood transfusion reactions
- Chemical agents
  - Lead
  - Sulfonamides
  - Antimalarial drugs
  - Analgesics
- Physical agents
  - Mechanical heart valve
  - Third-degree burns
- Infectious agents
  - Parasites
  - Bacteria

Recommended Actions
- Redraw specimens if hemolysis was caused by procedural error.

Partially Filled Tubes

Partially filled collection tubes deliver the wrong ratio of blood to anticoagulant, resulting in an inadequate specimen for laboratory testing. Examples of an incorrect ratio of blood to anticoagulant can result in the following:

- Excess liquid anticoagulant in light blue stopper tubes dilutes the plasma and causes prolonged coagulation testing.
- Excess ethylenediaminetraacetic acid (EDTA) in the lavender stopper tube shrinks the red blood cells and affects the hematocrit, red blood cell count, hemoglobin, red blood cell indices, and erythrocyte sedimentation rate (ESR) rates.
- Underfilled gray stopper tubes cause hemolysis of the red blood cells.
- Completely filled green stopper tubes are critical for ionized calcium tests.

Serum separator tubes (SST) and red stopper tubes are usually not affected by partially filled collection tubes, providing there is an adequate amount of specimen to perform the test.

Recommended Actions

- "Partial-draw" tubes are available for situations in which it is difficult to obtain a full tube. A line is present on each tube to indicate the proper fill level.

Specimen Rejection

Specimens brought to the laboratory may be rejected if conditions are present that would compromise the validity of the test results.

Common Reasons for Specimen Rejection

- Unlabeled or mislabeled specimens
- Inadequate volume
- Collection in the wrong tube
- Hemolysis
- Lipemia
- Clotted blood in an anticoagulant tube
- Improper handling during transport
- Missing requisition form
- Contaminated specimen containers

- Delays in specimen processing
- Use of outdated blood collection tubes

Recommended Actions
- Redraw the specimen.
- Always follow procedure and facility protocols.

Notes

_____

_____

_____

_____

_____

_____

_____

_____

_____

_____

_____

_____

_____

_____

_____

_____

_____

_____

Timed Specimens

Reasons for Timed Specimens
- Measure the body's ability to metabolize a particular substance
- Monitor changes in a patient's condition
- Determine blood levels of medications
- Measure substances that exhibit diurnal variation
- Measure cardiac markers after acute myocardial infarction
- Monitor anticoagulant therapy

Diurnal Variation

The levels of certain substances and cell counts in the blood change at different times of day. Therefore, specimens must be collected at specific times.

Major Analytes Affected by Diurnal Variation
- Corticosteroids
- Hormones
- Serum iron
- Glucose
- White blood cell count
- Eosinophil count
- Renin

🖑 **ALERT:** If the specimen cannot be collected at the specified time, notify the health-care provider.

Therapeutic Drug Monitoring

To ensure patient safety and medication effectiveness, many therapeutic drugs require monitoring of blood levels using the trough and peak level collection methods.

Frequently Monitored Therapeutic Drugs
- Amikacin
- Digoxin
- Dilantin
- Tobramycin
- Phenobarbital
- Gentamicin

- Lithium
- Theophylline
- Vancomycin
- Valproic acid
- Methotrexate
- Various antibiotics

Trough Levels
- Represent the lowest level in the blood
- Ensure the drug is within the therapeutic range
- Collected and tested immediately before the drug is to be administered

Peak Levels
- Represent the highest level in the blood
- Can be collected at different times, depending on the medication and method of administration

Examples
- 30 minutes after IV administration
- 60 minutes after intramuscular administration
- 1 to 2 hours after oral administration

🖐 **ALERT:** Follow the manufacturer's recommended times for collection of peak levels based on the half-life of the drug and toxicity level.

Oral Glucose Tolerance Tests (OGTTs)

OGTTs are performed to detect the presence of diabetes mellitus and gestational diabetes.

Patient Preparation
- Before the test, instruct the patient to eat a balanced diet that includes 150 g/day of carbohydrates for 3 days.
- Instruct the patient to abstain from food and drinks, except water, for 8 hours but not more than 16 hours before the test and during the test.
- Instruct the patient to avoid smoking, chewing tobacco, alcohol, sugarless gum, and vigorous exercise before and during the test.

Before the Test

🖐 **ALERT:** Before beginning the test, ask the patient about the use of substances that can interfere with test results, including alcohol, anticonvulsants, aspirin, birth control pills, blood pressure medications, corticosteroids, diuretics, and estrogen-replacement pills. Note their use on the requisition form or consult the health-care provider.

■ Collect and test a fasting glucose specimen, making sure to carefully check the health-care provider's orders before performing the test, because the amount of glucose given sometimes varies.

🖐 **ALERT:** Be aware of the need to collect and test a fasting glucose specimen before every OGTT to ensure that the patient can safely receive a large amount of glucose. Follow your facility's protocol.

OGTT PROCEDURE FOR DIABETES MELLITUS

Equipment
■ Requisition form
■ Requisition-specified glucose solution
■ Gloves
■ Tourniquet
■ Alcohol pads
■ Evacuated tube holder and needles
■ Evacuated tubes

🖐 **ALERT:** The type of evacuated tubes used for OGTT blood collection must be consistent.

■ 2-inch × 2-inch gauze
■ Sharps disposal container
■ Indelible pen
■ Bandage
■ Biohazard bag

🖐 **ALERT:** Collect blood specimens that will *not* be tested until the end of the OGTT in gray stopper tubes.

SPECIAL PROC

🖐 **ALERT:** Consistently use venipuncture or dermal puncture because glucose values differ between the two types of blood. Venous blood specimens are preferred.

Procedure

1. Obtain and examine the requisition form.
2. Identify the patient using the correct protocol and explain the procedure.
3. Confirm that the patient has fasted for 12 hours and not more than 16 hours.
4. Collect and test a fasting glucose specimen.
5. Instruct the patient to drink the entire amount of glucose solution within 5 minutes.

🖐 **ALERT:** Watch for changes in the patient's condition, such as dizziness, which might indicate a reaction to the glucose. Report any changes to a supervisor.

6. Begin timing the remaining collection times when the patient finishes drinking the glucose solution:
   - For an outpatient, provide a copy of the schedule and instruct the patient to continue fasting, to drink water, and to remain in the drawing station area.
   - For an inpatient, keep a copy of the schedule and go to the patient to collect the specimens at the specified times.

🖐 **ALERT:** If vomiting occurs, report the time of vomiting to a supervisor and contact the health-care provider to find out whether to continue the test. Vomiting early in the procedure is considered most critical and, in most situations, results in discontinuation of the OGTT.

7. Label the tubes with the specimen order in the test sequence, such as 1-hour, 2-hour, or 3-hour.

ONE-STEP METHOD FOR GESTATIONAL DIABETES

1. Administer a 75-g glucose challenge load to a patient who has fasted.

2. Collect blood at 1 and 2 hours after she drinks the 75-g glucose solution.
3. Deliver the labeled specimens to the laboratory.

TWO-STEP METHOD FOR GESTATIONAL DIABETES

The two-step method requires the patient to receive two tests. The second test should be administered on a different day.

Day 1

1. Administer a 50-g glucose challenge load to a nonfasting patient.
2. Collect blood 1 hour after the patient drinks the glucose solution.
3. Deliver the labeled specimen to the laboratory.

■ When the plasma glucose level is equal to or greater than 140 mg/dL, step 2 is performed.

Day 2

1. Administer a 100-g, 3-hour OGTT.
2. Collect blood specimens at the scheduled times after the patient finishes drinking the glucose solution.
3. Deliver the labeled specimens to the laboratory.

OGTT Notes

_____

_____

_____

_____

_____

_____

_____

_____

_____

_____

_____

_____

_____

Blood Cultures

✋ **ALERT:** Strict aseptic technique is required for the collection of blood cultures.

Timing and Sites of Blood Culture Collections
- Blood cultures are usually ordered routine, stat, or as timed collections.
- Specimens are collected in sets consisting of two bottles, one to be incubated aerobically and the other anaerobically.
- Collection of specimen sets from two different sites serves as a control of aseptic technique and aids in the recovery of microorganisms.
- Bottles should be labeled with the collection site and time of collection.

Examples of Collection Protocols
- Sets collected 30 to 60 minutes apart, each from a different site
- Sets collected just before a patient's temperature spikes
- Sets collected at the same time, each from a different site
- One set collected from an IV line and one set collected by venipuncture

✋ **ALERT:** Timing of collections varies. Follow the physician's orders and your facility's protocol.

Specialized Blood Culture Collection Equipment
- Bottles and tubes
  - Blood culture bottles contain culture media, the anticoagulant sodium polyanethol sulfonate (SPS), and a

81

vacuum to allow blood to be pulled directly into the bottle
during the venipuncture.

- Sterile, yellow stopper evacuated tubes contain SPS and
are used when the blood in the tube can be transferred at
a later time to a blood culture bottle in the laboratory.
- Winged blood collection sets attach to a specifically
designed holder for the blood culture bottles. This allows
the blood to be directly collected into the bottles.
- Sterile syringes and a safety transfer device can be used
to collect blood in a syringe and transfer it to a blood
culture bottle.
- Anticoagulants
  - The only acceptable anticoagulant for blood cultures is
  SPS. SPS is present in blood culture bottles and in yellow
  stopper evacuated tubes.

✋ ALERT: Be sure to gently invert both tubes and bottles eight
times to mix because bacteria can become trapped in a blood
clot and be unable to grow.

Cleansing the Site
- Strict aseptic technique is required when cleansing a
puncture site before collecting a blood culture.
- Blood cultures require the use of iodine or chlorhexidine
gluconate.

Using Iodine or Povidone Iodine
- Vigorously rub the site with isopropyl alcohol in a
back-and-forth motion for 1 minute.
- Scrub with iodine or povidone iodine in a back-and-forth
motion, progressing outward 3 to 4 inches for 1 minute.
- Allow the iodine to dry for at least 30 seconds.
- To prevent skin irritation, remove the iodine with isopropyl
alcohol when the procedure is finished.

Using Chlorhexidine Gluconate
- Using a commercially prepared swab or sponge
(ChloraPrep), vigorously rub the site for 30 to 60 seconds in
a back-and-forth motion, creating friction.

■ Allow the chlorhexidine gluconate to dry for at least 30 to 60 seconds.

🖐 **ALERT:** Be aware that contamination of blood culture bottles with normal skin bacteria can interfere with the interpretation of test results.

Cleansing the Blood Culture Bottle Tops
■ Cleanse the bottle tops using alcohol.

🖐 **ALERT:** Do not cleanse the tops with iodine because it can enter the bottle during inoculation and interfere with bacterial growth.

■ Allow the tops to dry.
■ Place a clean alcohol wipe over the tops until inoculation.

Specimen Collection
■ Collect two specimens for each blood culture set, one aerobic and one anaerobic.
  ■ When the specimen is collected using a syringe, inoculate the anaerobic bottle first to prevent possible exposure to air.
  ■ When the specimen is collected using a winged blood collection set, inoculate the aerobic bottle first so that the air in the tubing does not enter the anaerobic bottle and kill any anaerobic organisms present.

🖐 **ALERT:** The amount of blood inoculated into each container is critical. The ratio of blood to media should be at least 1:10. Adult blood culture bottles usually require 8 to 10 mL for each bottle, and pediatric bottles require 1 to 3 mL for each bottle. Read the bottle label for the volume of blood required.

BLOOD CULTURE PROCEDURE

Equipment
■ Requisition form
■ Gloves
■ Tourniquet

■ Acceptable blood culture skin antiseptic
■ Alcohol pads

83

- Blood culture bottles
- 2-inch × 2-inch gauze
- Sharps disposal container
- Indelible pen
- Bandage

OR

- Syringe, hypodermic needle with safety device or Point-Lok device, and blood transfer device

- Winged blood collection set and tube holder

Procedure

1. Obtain and examine the requisition form.
2. Greet, identify the patient using the correct protocol, and explain the procedure to be performed.
3. Select equipment.

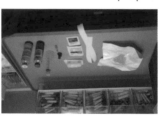

4. Sanitize your hands.
5. Put on gloves.
6. Apply a tourniquet.
7. Locate a venipuncture site.
8. Release the tourniquet.
9. Disinfect the site using the correct blood culture cleansing method.

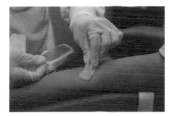

10. Assemble the equipment while the antiseptic is drying.
11. Remove the plastic cap from each collection bottle.
12. Confirm the volume of blood required from each label.

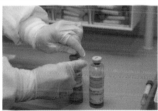

13. Clean the top of each bottle with a 70% isopropyl alcohol pad and then allow it to dry.

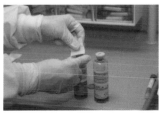

14. Reapply the tourniquet.
15. Perform the venipuncture.

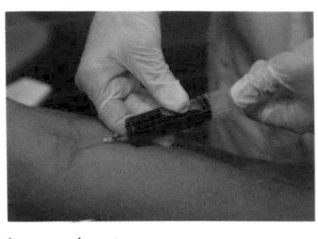

16. Release the tourniquet.
17. Place gauze over the puncture site, remove the needle, and apply pressure.
18. Activate the safety device or remove the syringe needle with a Point-Lok device.

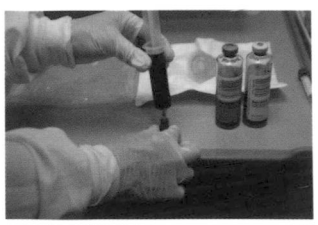

19. Immediately dispose of the needle or syringe in a sharps disposal container.
20. Attach a safety transfer device.

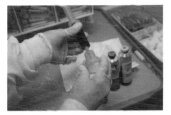

21. Inoculate the anaerobic blood culture bottle first when using the syringe and second when using a winged blood collection set.

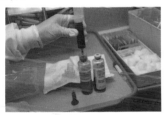

22. Dispense the correct amount of blood into the bottles and document the amount if required by the facility.
23. Mix the blood culture bottles by gently inverting them eight times.
24. If other tests are ordered, fill the other collection tubes after the blood culture tubes according to the order of draw.
25. Clean the iodine off the patient's arm with alcohol.

26. Label the specimens appropriately, including the site of collection, their number in the series, and time of collection. Verify the identification with the patient.
27. Dispose of used supplies.
28. Check the venipuncture site for bleeding.
29. Bandage the patient's arm.
30. Thank the patient.
31. Remove your gloves.
32. Sanitize your hands.

Blood Culture Notes

Special Specimen Handling Procedures

The levels of certain analytes can change if correct specimen handling procedures are not followed.

Specimens That Must Be Kept at Body Temperature

- Cold agglutinins are antibodies that, when blood cools, attach to red blood cells and can no longer be measured in the serum.
- Cryofibrinogen and cryoglobulin are proteins that precipitate when blood cools.

Procedure
- Obtain a collection tube that has been warmed at 37°C for 30 minutes.
- Transport the tube to the patient in a portable warmer.
- Collect the specimen as quickly as possible.
- Return it to the laboratory in a warmer or tightly closed fist.
- Place the specimen in a 37°C incubator until testing.

Specimens That Must Be Chilled

- Acetone
- Adrenocorticotropic hormone
- Ammonia
- Angiotensin-converting enzyme
- Arterial blood gases (if not tested within 30 minutes)
- Catecholamines
- Free fatty acids
- Gastrin
- Glucagon
- Homocysteine
- Lactic acid
- Parathyroid hormone
- Pyruvate
- Renin
- Some coagulation studies

💧 **ALERT:** Do not chill specimens unless indicated in the procedure as a part of specimen processing.

Procedure

■ Place the specimen in crushed ice, an ice slurry (mixture of ice and water), or a temperature-controlled ice block.

✋ ALERT: Do not place the specimen in or on large ice cubes because part of it may freeze.

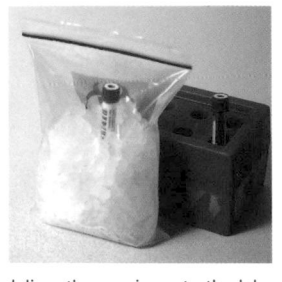

■ Immediately deliver the specimen to the laboratory.

✋ ALERT: Never chill specimens that are to be tested for electrolytes and prothrombin times. Arterial specimens for blood gases analysis collected in plastic syringes are not chilled but must be tested within 30 minutes.

Specimens That Are Sensitive to Light

■ Beta-carotene
■ Bilirubin
■ Folate
■ Porphyrins

■ Vitamin A
■ Vitamin B_6
■ Vitamin B_{12}

Procedure

■ Collect the specimen in an amber-colored container or wrap the specimen in aluminum foil.

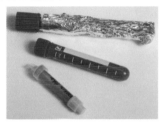

Specimen Storage

To prevent contamination of plasma and serum by cellular constituents, it is recommended that specimens be separated within 2 hours. Anticoagulated specimens can be centrifuged immediately after collection, and the plasma removed. Specimens collected without anticoagulant must be fully clotted before centrifugation. Specimens for hematology whole blood analysis should never be centrifuged.

Based on the tests requested, separated serum or plasma may remain at room temperature for 8 hours. If testing has not been completed in 8 hours, the sample should be refrigerated. If testing is not complete in 48 hours, the serum or plasma should be frozen. Refer to the procedure manual for specific analyte instructions.

CLSI recommends time limits for testing of specimens. Examples include the following:

■ Coagulation specimens for activated partial thromboplastin times (APTTs) are stable at room temperature for 4 hours unless the patient is on heparin, in which case the plasma must be removed from the cells within 1 hour after collection and tested within 4 hours.

- Specimens for prothrombin time (PT) testing are stable for 24 hours at room temperature.
- All other coagulation tests must be performed within 4 hours of collection. When specimens cannot be assayed within the required time frame, the platelet-poor plasma must be separated from the red cells and frozen within 1 hour of collection.
- Blood smears from EDTA tubes must be made within 1 hour of collection to avoid cell distortion and artifact caused by the EDTA anticoagulant.
- EDTA samples for CBCs are stable for 24 hours at room temperature; however, for certain manufacturer's tubes, CBCs should be analyzed within 6 hours. EDTA specimens for CBCs collected in microcollection containers must be tested in 4 hours.
- ESR tests must be performed within 4 hours in EDTA specimens stored at room temperature or within 12 hours when refrigerated.
- Reticulocyte counts collected in EDTA should be analyzed within 6 hours when stored at room temperature or up to 72 hours when refrigerated.
- Specimens for glucose tests collected in sodium fluoride tubes are stable for 24 hours at room temperature and 48 hours when refrigerated.

Legal (Forensic) Specimens

Documentation of specimen handling, called the *chain of custody* (COC), is essential.

- Chain of custody begins with patient identification and continues until testing is completed and the results are reported.
- Special forms are provided for this documentation, and special containers and seals may be required.
- Each person handling the specimen must document the date, time, and his or her personal identification.
- Patient identification and specimen collection should be done in the presence of a witness.

SPECIAL
PROC

🖐 **ALERT:** Technical errors and failure to follow chain-of-custody protocol are primary defense targets in legal proceedings.

Blood Alcohol Specimens

■ Clean the site with soap and water or a nonalcoholic antiseptic solution.

🖐 **ALERT:** Do not use alcohol to clean the site because it compromises the results.

■ To prevent the escape of the volatile alcohol, completely fill tubes and do not uncap.
■ Collect specimens in gray stopper tubes or tubes specified by the laboratory. Check laboratory protocol.

Specimens for DNA Testing

■ Be aware that paternity tests may require finger or heel printing for identification.
■ Although yellow stopper acid citrate dextrose (ACD) tubes are commonly used for blood analysis, check with the laboratory because two different concentrations of ACD are available, and other specialized tubes may be required based on the test procedure in use.

Urine Specimens for Drug Testing

For urine specimens to withstand legal scrutiny, it is necessary to prove that no tampering (e.g., adulteration, substitution, or dilution) took place.

Collection Procedure

1. Sanitize hands and put on gloves.
2. Add bluing agent (dye) to the toilet water reservoir to prevent an adulterated specimen.
3. Eliminate any source of water other than toilet by taping the toilet lid and faucet handles.
4. Have the donor provide photo identification or obtain positive identification from an employer representative.
5. Complete step 1 of the COC form and have the donor sign the form.

6. Have the donor leave any personal belongings (e.g., coat, briefcase, purse) outside the collection area to avoid the possibility of concealed substances contaminating the urine.

7. Have the donor wash his or her hands.

8. Give the donor a specimen cup.

9. Remain in the restroom but outside the stall, listening for unauthorized water use, unless a witnessed collection is requested.

10. Have the donor hand the specimen cup to you.

11. Check the urine for abnormal color and for the required amount (30 to 45 mL).

12. Check that the temperature strip on the specimen cup reads between 32.5°C and 37.7°C. If it does, record the temperature on the COC form (COC step 2). If the specimen temperature is out of range or if you suspect that the specimen has been diluted or adulterated, collect a new specimen and notify a supervisor.

13. Keep the specimen in your sight and the donor's sight at all times.

14. With the donor watching, peel off the specimen identification strips from the COC form (COC step 3) and put them on the capped bottle, covering both sides of the cap.

15. Ask the donor to initial the specimen bottle seals.

16. Write the date and time on the seals.

17. Complete steps 4 and 5 on the COC form.

🖐 **ALERT:** Each time the specimen is handled, transferred, or placed in storage, every individual must be identified and the date and purpose of the change recorded.

18. Follow laboratory-specific instructions for packaging the specimen bottles and laboratory copies of the COC form.

19. Distribute the COC copies to appropriate personnel.

Special Handling Notes

_____

_____

_____

_____

_____

_____

_____

_____

_____

_____

_____

_____

_____

Blood Collection From Vascular Access Devices

General Considerations

■ Specimens can only be collected from central venous catheters (CVCs) and vascular access devices (VADs) by personnel who have received **specialized training in the procedures.**

■ Numerous types of CVCs and VADs exist, and specific procedures must be followed for flushing the catheters with

saline solution, and possibly heparin to prevent thrombosis, when blood collection is completed.

■ Sterile technique must be strictly adhered to when entering IV lines because they provide a direct path for infectious organisms to enter a patient's bloodstream.

■ When IV fluids are being administered through a CVC, the flow should be stopped for 1 minute before collecting the blood specimen.

■ Syringes larger than 20 mL should not be used because the high negative pressure produced may collapse the catheter wall.

■ At all times, the first 5 mL of blood (or two times the dead space volume of the catheter) must be discarded and a new syringe must be used to collect the specimen.

■ Drawing coagulation tests from a venous catheter is not recommended but, if necessary, should be performed only after 20 mL (or five to six times the dead space volume of the catheter) of blood have been discarded or used for other tests.

Order of Fill

When Blood Cultures Are Ordered

1. First syringe: 5 mL discard
2. Second syringe: Blood cultures
3. Third syringe:
   a. Anticoagulated specimens
   b. Clotted specimens

When Blood Cultures Are Not Ordered

1. First syringe: 5 mL discard
2. Second syringe: All specimens except coagulation specimens
3. Third syringe: Coagulation specimens

COLLECTION PROCEDURE USING A CVC

Equipment

- Requisition form
- Gloves
- Alcohol wipes or chlorhexidine gluconate sponge
- Two 10-mL syringes filled with normal saline solution (for flush)
- Two 5-mL syringes
- Three-way stopcock
- Blood collection tubes
- Syringes for blood collection
- Blood transfer device
- One or two 5 mL syringe(s) filled with heparinized saline for flushing after using the saline flush (optional)

Procedure

1. Obtain and examine the requisition form.
2. Verify the patient's identity using two identifiers.
3. Explain the procedure and obtain patient's informed consent.
4. Position the patient in a supine position.
5. Assemble the supplies.
6. Sanitize your hands and put on gloves.
7. Stop infusions in all lumens for 1 minute before drawing the specimen. When the lumen to be used for laboratory draws has an infusion, cap the tubing with a male/female cap when disconnecting it.
8. When drawing from multilumen catheters, clamp all lumens and withdraw blood from the proximal lumen of the catheter.
9. Cleanse the injection cap with an alcohol wipe. Using vigorous friction, scrub on the top and in the grooves for 15 seconds. When the laboratory draw is for a blood culture, scrub the injection cap with an alcohol wipe for 30 seconds.

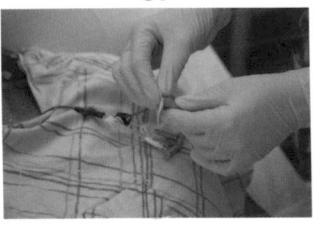

10. Attach a 10-mL prefilled saline syringe to a three-way stopcock. Flush with 10 mL of normal saline (if TPN or heparin was infusing, flush the line with 20 mL of normal saline).

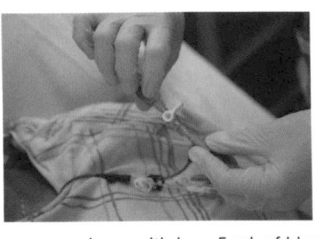

11. Using the same syringe, withdraw 5 mL of blood. Remove the syringe and discard the syringe in a biohazard container. Wait 10 to 15 seconds to draw the specimen.

🖐 **ALERT:** Flush the CVCs to ensure and maintain the patency of the catheter and to prevent mixing of medications and solutions that are incompatible. Follow the manufacturer's instructions for correct use and your facility's policy and procedure for flushing. Incomplete flushing of the collection site can cause contamination or dilution of the specimen, causing errors in test results.

12. Use a sterile syringe to collect the specimen. **Collect the smallest volume of blood required for each test.**

13. Attach the syringe and blood collection tubes to the blood transfer device and fill the tubes in the correct order

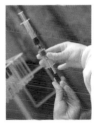

14. After the tubes are filled, mix them immediately by gentle inversion for the appropriate number of inversions.
15. Label all tubes in front of the patient and confirm with the patient or the identification (ID) band that the information is correct.
16. Scrub the hub for 15 seconds with alcohol to remove any blood.
17. Attach a prefilled, nonsterile 10-mL saline syringe and flush. Use two syringes for a total of 20 mL. If there are lumens that are not being used, flush each of these lumens with 10 mL of saline.

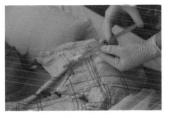

18. Resume previous fluids if applicable.

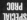

BLOOD COLLECTION FROM AN IMPLANTED PORT

Equipment

- Requisition form
- Sterile drape
- Sterile gloves
- Noncoring needle
- Two 10-mL syringes
- Two 10-mL flush syringes filled with saline
- One 10-mL syringe filled with heparinized flush solution (follow facility protocol)
- Chlorhexidine gluconate sponge or alcohol and iodine pads
- One 5-mL syringe
- 2-inch × 2-inch gauze pads
- Dressing to cover insertion site

Procedure

1. Obtain and review the requisition form.
2. Identify the patient verbally by having him or her state both the first and last names, spell the last name, and give the date of birth. Compare the information on the patient's identification (ID) band with the requisition form.
3. Explain the procedure, and obtain the patient's informed consent.
4. Sanitize your hands, and put on sterile gloves.
5. Assemble your equipment.
6. Palpate the patient's shoulder area to locate and identify the septum of the access port.
7. Prep the area with a vigorous scrub using a chlorhexidine gluconate applicator. When using alcohol and iodine pads, prep in a circular motion from within to outward, approximately 4 to 6 inches, first with the alcohol pad and and

19. Prepare the specimen and requisition form for transport to the laboratory.
20. Dispose of used supplies in a biohazard container.
21. Remove your gloves, sanitize your hands, and thank the patient.

then with the iodine swab. Allow the disinfectant to dry completely (30 to 60 seconds for antisepsis to occur).

8. Connect the noncoring needle tubing on the end of one 10-mL saline flush syringe, and prime the needle with saline until it is expelled.

9. Locate the septum of the port with your nondominant hand; firmly anchor the port between your thumb and forefinger.

10. Holding the noncoring needle with your other hand, puncture the patient's skin and insert the needle at a 90-degree angle into the septum using firm pressure. Advance the needle until resistance is met and the needle touches the back wall of the port.

11. Inject 1 to 2 mL of saline, and observe the area for swelling and ease of flow; if swelling occurs, reposition the needle in the port without withdrawing it from the skin. If there is not swelling, aspirate for blood return. When blood return is observed, continue to flush with saline.

12. Using the same syringe, aspirate 10 mL of blood, and discard it. When specimens will be collected for coagulation studies, discard 20 mL.

13. Attach the syringe or the evacuated tube holder to the needle tubing, and collect the **minimum** blood necessary for ordered laboratory tests.

14. Dispense the blood into the appropriate blood collection tubes (using a blood transfer device when a syringe is used) in the correct order of fill. Mix the blood by gentle inversion three to eight times.

15. Flush the needle and the port with 20 mL of saline.

16. Change syringes, and flush with 3 mL of heparinized saline or follow your facility's policy.

17. Remove the needle, and apply a sterile dressing over the site.

18. Label all tubes in front of the patient, and confirm with the patient or ID band that the information is correct.

19. Prepare the specimen and requisition form for transport to the laboratory.

20. Dispose of used supplies in the appropriate biohazard container.

21. Remove your gloves, sanitize your hands, and thank the patient.

🖑 **ALERT:** Always wear sterile gloves when accessing ports. Maintain sterile technique throughout the procedure.

🖑 **ALERT:** Be aware that potential test errors can occur with blood obtained from VADs due to hemolysis caused by air leaks when using incompatible blood collection components.

🖑 **ALERT:** Be aware that inadequate flushing of the collection site can contaminate or dilute the specimen and cause erroneous test results.

CVC and VAD Notes

_____

_____

_____

_____

_____

_____

_____

_____

_____

_____

_____

_____

Urine Collection

Types of Urine Specimens
- Random specimens are collected at any time for routine urinalysis.
- First morning specimens are collected as soon as the patient arises and are used for confirmation of routine urinalysis, pregnancy testing, and orthostatic proteinuria.
- Clean-catch midstream specimens are collected for urine cultures.
- Catheterized specimens are collected from the bladder under sterile conditions for cultures.
- Suprapubic aspirations collect urine from the bladder externally for cultures and cytological examination.

Clean Catch Midstream Urine Collection for Women

Equipment
- Requisition form
- Sterile urine container with label
- Sterile antiseptic towelettes
- Written instructions for cleansing and voiding

Patient Instructions
1. Sanitize your hands.
2. Remove the lid from the container without touching the inside of the container or lid.
3. Separate the skin folds (labia).
4. Cleanse from front to back on either side of the urinary opening with an antiseptic towelette, using a clean one for each side.
5. Holding the skin folds apart, begin to void into the toilet.
6. Bring the urine container into the stream of urine and collect an adequate amount.

✋ **ALERT:** Do not touch the inside of the container or allow the container to touch the genital area.

7. Finish voiding into the toilet.
8. Cover the specimen with the lid, touching only the outside of the lid and container.
9. Label the container with your name and time of collection, and place it in the specified area or hand it to the collector for labeling.

Clean Catch Midstream Urine Collection Procedure for Men

Equipment
- Requisition form
- Sterile urine container with label
- Sterile antiseptic towelettes
- Written instructions for cleansing and voiding

Patient Instructions
1. Sanitize your hands.
2. Remove the lid from the sterile container without touching the inside of the container or lid.
3. Cleanse the tip of the penis with an antiseptic towelette and let it dry. Retract the foreskin if uncircumcised.
4. Void into the toilet, holding back the foreskin if necessary.
5. Bring the sterile urine container into the stream of urine and collect an adequate amount.

✋ **ALERT:** Do not touch the inside of the container or allow the container to touch the genital area.

6. Finish voiding into the toilet.
7. Cover the specimen with the lid, touching only the outside of the lid and container.
8. Label the container with your name and the time of collection, and place it in the specified area or hand it to the collector for labeling.

24-Hour (Timed) Urine Specimen Collection

■ Used for quantitative measurement of urine constituents
■ To obtain an accurate timed specimen, the patient must begin and end the collection period with an empty bladder.

Equipment

■ Requisition form
■ 24-hour urine specimen container with lid
■ Label
■ Container with ice, if required
■ Preservative, if required

Procedure

1. Explain the collection procedure, and provide the patient with written instructions.
2. Issue the proper collection container and preservative.
3. **Day 1:** The patient voids and discards first morning specimen.
4. The patient writes the exact time on the specimen label and places the label on the container.
5. The patient collects all subsequent urine for the next 24 hours.

✋ **ALERT:** The patient should collect any urine specimen before any bowel movement to avoid fecal contamination.

✋ **ALERT:** The patient should refrigerate the specimen after adding each urine collection.

6. The patient should continue to drink normal amounts of fluid throughout the collection time.
7. **Day 2:** The patient voids and adds the first morning urine to the previously collected urine.
8. The patient transports the specimen to the laboratory in an insulated bag or portable cooler.
9. The entire 24-hour specimen is thoroughly mixed in the laboratory, and the volume is accurately measured and recorded.
10. A sufficient aliquot is saved for testing and possible additional testing.
11. The remaining urine is discarded.

Urine Collection Notes

_____

_____

_____

_____

_____

_____

_____

_____

_____

_____

_____

_____

_____

_____

_____

_____

_____

_____

Throat Culture Collection

- Specimens may be collected for the purpose of performing a culture or a rapid immunological group A strep test.

SPECIAL PROC

THROAT CULTURE SPECIMEN COLLECTION PROCEDURE

Equipment
- Requisition form
- Tongue depressor
- Collection swab(s) in a sterile tube containing transport media
- Flashlight

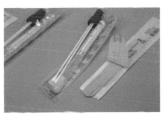

Procedure
1. Obtain and examine the requisition form.
2. Identify the patient using the correct protocol.
3. Sanitize your hands.
4. Put on gloves.
5. Ask the patient to tilt the head back and open the mouth wide.
6. Remove the cap with its attached swab(s) from the tube using sterile technique.

👆 ALERT: If necessary, use a flashlight to illuminate the back of the throat.

7. Gently depress the tongue with the tongue depressor, and ask the patient to say "ah."

8. Being careful not to touch the cheeks, tongue, or lips, swab the area in the back of the throat, including the tonsils, and any inflamed or ulcerated areas.

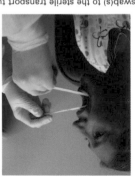

9. Return the swab(s) to the sterile transport tube.

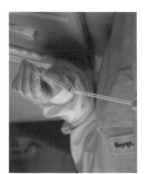

10. Close the cap.

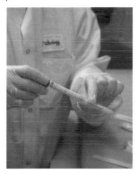

11. Crush the ampule of transport medium (if necessary), making sure the released medium is in contact with the swabs.

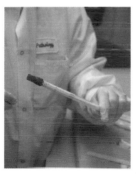

12. Label the specimen.
13. Remove your gloves.
14. Sanitize your hands.
15. Immediately deliver the specimen to the microbiology laboratory.

Throat Culture Collection Notes

_____

_____

_____

_____

_____

_____

_____

_____

_____

_____

_____

_____

_____

_____

_____

_____

Point of Care Testing (POCT)

Specimens for POCT can be collected by dermal puncture and tested in the patient area.

POCT Procedures Commonly Collected by Dermal Puncture

- Glucose testing
- Hgb A1c
- Hemoglobin testing
- Cholesterol testing
- Microhematocrit testing
- Infectious mononucleosis testing
- Coagulation testing

✋ **ALERT:** POCT coagulation tests commonly specify to use the first drop of blood obtained by dermal puncture for testing.

✋ **ALERT:** Tests are continually being developed and added to the waived test category. For an up-to-date listing of waived tests, refer to https://www.cms.gov/Regulations-and-Guidance/Legislation/CLIA/Downloads/waivetbl.pdf.

Prevention of Errors in POCT

- Patient identification
  - Identify the correct patient.
  - Use the patient's full name and a second identifier on all specimens, requisition forms, and reports.
- Proper specimen collection
  - Ensure the correct specimen type is collected.
  - Use the correct collection technique.
  - Label all specimens.
  - Handle and transport specimens according to procedure.
- Proper storage of testing supplies
  - Store reagents at the correct storage temperature.
  - Never use an expired test reagent or collection device.

- Quality control (QC)
  - Perform and document QC according to the procedure and your facility's protocol.
  - Always confirm that QC results are within the expected range before performing or reporting any patient testing.
- Specimen application and test performance
  - Always follow the manufacturer's instructions for applying the specimen to the test device.
  - Strictly follow test-timing instructions.
- Result interpretation
  - Refer to the test procedure for correct interpretation of test results, confirmatory testing that may be required, and guidance for identification and communication of critical results.
- Documentation of results
  - Record results in the permanent medical record so that they are legible and easily retrieved.

Common Errors Associated With POCT

Tests	Errors
Coagulation tests	• Failure to adequately cleanse and dry the capillary puncture site • Failure to follow the manufacturer's instructions for specimen collection • Premature capillary puncture before the test strip or cartridge is ready to accept the specimen • Inadequate specimen application

Continued

Tests	Errors
Glucose	• Use of compromised or expired reagent strips • Failure to adequately cleanse and dry the capillary puncture site • Failure to adequately or correctly apply specimen to testing area • Failure to run controls and document as required
Group A *Streptococcus*	• Use of cotton or calcium alginate collection swabs • Use of compromised or expired reagent kits • Failure to observe the internal control • Incorrect collection or timing
Hemoglobin	• Failure to adequately fill the cuvette • Bubbles in the cuvette
Immunoassay kits	• Use of reagents from different kits • Failure to follow the step-by-step instructions • Use of incorrectly stored or expired kits • Misinterpretation of test and control results • Failure to observe and document internal control results
i-STAT profiles	• Failure to correctly identify the patient in the meter • Failure to observe cartridge warm-up time • Failure to comply with room temperature expiration dates • Return of room temperature cartridges to refrigerated storage • Underfilling or overfilling of cartridges • Squeezing of a closed cartridge • Device movement during analysis of specimen • Failure to upload the meter for timely data transfer

Continued

Tests	Errors
Occult blood (guaiac slide methods)	• Failure to allow the specimen to dry on the testing area prior to adding the reagent • Failure to provide patient with precollection instructions • Failure to use the correct specimen type for the test • Failure to apply the correct amount of specimen on the slide • Failure to wait the specified time after the specimen is applied to add the developer reagent
POC meters (analyzers with data management)	• Failure to correctly identify the patient in the meter • Failure to follow correct timing for application of the specimen to the test strip or cartridge • Failure to follow correct timing for placing the test strip or cartridge in the meter • Failure to upload the meter for timely data transfer
Toxicology profile	• Use of incorrectly stored or expired kits • Misinterpretation of patient and control results
Urinalysis	• Use of compromised or expired reagent strips • Incorrect reaction timing • Failure to follow correct timing (i.e., leaving the reagent strips in the specimen for too long)
Urine pregnancy test	• Failure to test a first morning specimen • Addition of reagents in the wrong order • Misinterpretation of test and control results

POCT Notes

Antidiuretic hormone test, 174

Antiglycolytic agent, as additive, 7

Anti–hepatitis A virus test, 174

Anti–hepatitis B surface antigen test, 174

Anti–hepatitis C virus test, 174

Anti-HIV test, 174

Antinuclear antibody test, 175

Antistreptolysin O titer, 175

Antithrombin III test, 175

Antiviral agents, after HIV exposure, 168

Apolipoprotein tests, 175

Arm veins
anchoring of, 35
palpation of, 34
patient positioning and, 29
selection of, 26

Arterial puncture, 140–156
for arterial blood gas testing, 140–156
artery selection criteria for, 142
complications of, 153, 155–156
errors in, 154–155
local anesthetic in, 146–147
modified Allen test before, 143–145
patient assessment in, 141
pressure application after, 151–152
procedure for radial, 148–153
site preparation in, 146
site selection in, 142–145
specimen integrity in, 154
as venipuncture complication, 69

Aseptic technique, for blood cultures, 80

Aspartate aminotransferase test, 175

Aspirin
laboratory tests and, 60
test for, 187

Assay. *See specific assay.*

B

Bacillus, alcohol-based cleansers and, 157

Bacterial infections, isolation precautions for, 162–164

Bandage
after dermal puncture, 122
after venipuncture, 41–42, 48
contraindication of, in young children, 128, 133

Base excess or deficit test, 140

Basic metabolic panel, 175

BD Vacutainer collection tubes, 8–11

Beta human chorionic gonadotropin, 175

Beta-carotene test, 177

Bicarbonate test, 140

Bilirubin tests
description of, 175
newborn, 119

Biohazard containers, for sharps disposal, 5

Blood
postexposure protocol for, 167–168
procedure for cleanup of, 166

Blood alcohol specimen procedure, 92

Blood collection. *See also specific procedures*
  equipment for, 1–24. *See also* Equipment; *specific equipment*
  failure to obtain blood. *See* Failure to obtain blood
  from implanted port, 99–101
Blood collection tubes, 6–15
  additives in, 6–14
  BD Vacutainer, 8–11
  centrifugation recommendations for, 14
  closures for, 8–13
  CLSI order of draw when using, 15
  inversion of, 40, 47, 54
  labeling of, 6, 41, 47
  laboratory uses of, 8–11
  mixing of, 40, 47, 54
  overview of, 8–13
  stoppers for, 8–13
  Vacuette, 12–14
Blood cultures, 80–87
  aerobic and anaerobic specimens for, 82, 86
  central venous catheter collection for, 96
  equipment for, 80–81
  overview of, 176
  procedure for, 82–87
  protocol examples for, 80
  site cleansing for, 81–82
  specimen amount for, 82
  timing and sites of, 80
Blood gas collection
  arterial, 140–156
  capillary, 130–133
  by heel puncture, 130–133

Blood group and type testing, 176
Blood pressure cuffs, as tourniquets, 32
Blood smear preparation
  equipment for, 134
  procedure for, 135–138
Blood tests, after blood and body fluid exposure, 167
Blood transfer device, 20–21
Blood urea nitrogen test, 176
Blow drying of slides, red blood cells distortion from, 137
Blunting device, needle, 2
Body fluids
  postexposure protocol for, 167–168
  procedure for cleanup of, 166
Body temperature specimens, 88
Bottles, for blood culture, 80–81
Brain natriuretic protein test, 170
Burned skin, venipuncture avoided in, 27

C
C3, 186
C4, 186
CA 125, 177
Caffeine, as laboratory test variable, 56
Calcitonin test, 176
Calcium test, 176, 183
Cancer antigen test, 177
Capillary blood gas collection
  equipment for, 130
  procedure for, 130–133
Carbamazepine (Tegretol) test, 177
Carbon monoxide test, 177

Carcinoembryonic antigen test, 177

Catheterized urine specimens from bladder, 102

Centers for Disease Control and Prevention
handwashing guidelines of, 157
immunizations recommended by, 158

Central venous catheter and access collection
blood collection from, 94–101
equipment for, 96
order of fill in, 95
overview of, 94–95
procedure for, 96–99

Centrifugation, of collection tubes, 14

Chain of custody
for forensic specimens, 91–92
for urine drug tests, 93

Chemical precautions, 169

Chemistry panels, 177

Chemotherapy, laboratory tests and, 60

Chickenpox immunization, 158

Chilled specimens
of arterial blood, 154
handling of, 88–89

Chlorhexidine
for arterial puncture, 146
for blood culture collection, 81–82
uses of, 22

Cholesterol test, 177

Cholesterol-lowering drugs, laboratory tests and, 60

Chromium test, 177

Citrate, as additive, 6

Cleansing of site
in arterial puncture procedure, 146
for blood alcohol specimens, 92
for blood culture collection, 81–82
in venipuncture procedure, 37, 44, 50

Clinical and Laboratory Standards Institute (CLSI)
arterial blood specimen recommendations of, 154
order of draw recommended by, 15
second phlebotomist mandated by, 65
specimen testing time limits, 90–91

Clostridium difficile, alcohol-based cleansers and, 157

Clot activators, as additives, 7

Coagulation specimens, 90

Coagulation tests
central venous catheter collection for, 95
dermal puncture protocol for, 110
errors in, 111

Cold agglutinins
special handling of, 88
test for, 177

Compartment syndrome, as venipuncture complication, 69

Complement level testing, 178

Complete blood count, 91, 178

Complications, 56–74. *See also specific complications*
  arterial puncture, 69, 153, 155–156
  dietary supplements and, 62
  errors affecting patients as, 67–69
  errors affecting specimens as, 70–74
  failure to obtain blood as, 63–65
  glucose tolerance tests, 78
  medications and, 60–61
  patient-related, 65–67
  pre-examination variables and, 56–60

Comprehensive metabolic panel, 177

Contact transmission, infection control precautions in, 164

Contamination prevention, in urine drug testing, 93

Copper test, 178

Corticosteroids, laboratory tests and, 61

Cortisol test, 178

C-peptide test, 176

C-reactive protein test, 178

Creatine kinase tests, 178

Creatinine test, 178

Crossmatch, 178

Cryofibrinogen, 88

Cryoglobulin
  special handling of, 88
  test for, 178

Cyclosporine test, 179

D

D-dimer test, 179

Dehydration, as laboratory test variable, 57

Delayed analysis, arterial blood gas test errors from, 155

Dermal puncture
  for blood smear collection, 134–138
  in capillary blood gas collection, 130–133
  equipment for, 117–118
  for glucose tolerance tests, 78
  in newborn screening, 125–128
  for point of care testing, 110
  procedure for, 118–122
  sites for, 115–116

Diabetes mellitus, glucose tolerance tests for, 76–80

Dietary supplements, coagulation and, 62

Differential blood count, 179

Digoxin test, 179

Direct antihuman globulin test, 179

Direct Coombs test, 179

Discard tube, 54

Disseminated intravascular coagulation panel, 179

Diuretics, laboratory tests and, 61

Diurnal variation
  analytes affected by, 75
  as laboratory test variable, 57

DNA testing specimen collection, 92

Droplet transmission, infection control precautions in, 163

Drug monitoring, therapeutic,
75-76
Drug screen, 179
Drug testing, urine specimens
for, 92-93

E

Earlobes, as contraindicated
dermal puncture sites, 116
EDTA
as additive, 6, 17
blood smears from, 91
in partially filled tubes, 73
specimen chilling
contraindicated for, 89
Electrolytes
Epstein-Barr virus panel, 179
tests of, 179
Equipment
for arterial puncture, 146, 148
for blood culture collection,
80-81
for blood smear preparation,
134
blood transfer device as,
20-21
for capillary blood gas
collection, 20-21
for central venous catheter
collection, 130
chart for location of, 172
collection, 96
collection tubes as, 6-15
for dermal puncture, 117-118
in evacuated tube system, 1,
35-36
fire extinguisher as, 171
needle holders as, 4
needles as, 1-3. See also
Needle(s)

for newborn screening, 125
order of draw and, 15-16
personal protective, 159-162
quality control in, 23
sharps disposal containers
as, 5
in syringe system, 20, 43
for throat culture collection,
106
tourniquets as, 31
in winged blood collection
sets, 21-22, 49
Errors
from arterial blood gas
specimen handling,
154-155
in arterial puncture,
154-155
patient-affecting
venipuncture, 67-69
in point of care testing,
110-113
specimen-affecting
venipuncture, 70-74
Erythrocyte sedimentation rate,
73, 179
Estrogen, laboratory tests and,
61
Ethanol/alcohol test, 180
Evacuate, in fire protocol, 171
Evacuated tube system
additives in, 6-14
blood transfer device for,
20-21
components of, 1, 35-36
for glucose tolerance tests, 77
labeling of, 6
venipuncture using, 35-42
in winged blood collection
sets, 22

Exercise
  as contraindicated before
    blood gas tests, 141
  as laboratory test variable,
    57–58
Expiration dates, in quality
  control, 23
Explosion and fire precautions,
  171
Extinguish, in fire protocol, 171

F

Factor assays, 180
Failure to obtain blood
  poor puncture device
    placement in, 120, 126, 135,
    138
  as venipuncture complication,
    63–65
Fainting, as venipuncture
  complication, 65–66
Fasting
  for glucose tolerance tests, 76
  as laboratory test variable, 58
Febrile antibody panel, 180
Femoral artery puncture,
  personnel restrictions for, 142
Ferritin test, 180
Fibrin degradation product test,
  180
Fibrinogen test, 180
Filter paper, in newborn
  screening, 126–128
Finger puncture
  in blood smear collection,
    135–136
  as contraindicated in young
    infants, 116
  patient positioning for, 118

procedure for, 118–122
sites for, 116
Fire and explosion precautions,
  171
First morning urine specimens,
  102
Flat arm support, for
  venipuncture, 30
Fluorescein dye, laboratory
  tests and, 61
Fluorescent antinuclear
  antibody test, 180
Fluorescent treponemal
  antibody-absorption test, 181
Flushing, of central venous
  catheters, 97
Folate test, 181
Forensic specimen handling,
  91–93
Free T$_4$, 187

G

G6PD test. See Glucose-6-
  phosphate dehdrogenase
  test.
Galactosemia screening, in
  newborns, 125
Gamma-glutamyl
  transpeptidase test, 181
Gangrene, as arterial puncture
  complication, 156
Gastrin test, 181
Gestational diabetes, glucose
  tolerance tests for, 78–79
Gloves
  for accessing ports, 101
  donning of, 160–161
  indications for, 159
  removal of, 161–162

for unfixed slide handling, 138
in venipuncture procedure,
25, 35–36, 44, 49–50
Glucose tests
errors in, 112
overview of, 181
Glucose tolerance tests, 76–80
dermal puncture for, 78
for diabetes mellitus, 76–80
equipment for, 77
for gestational diabetes,
78–79
interaction avoidance, 76–77
preparation for, 76–77
Glucose-6-phosphate
dehydrogenase (G6PD) test,
181
Goggles, 159
Gowns
donning of, 161
removal of, 162
requirements for, 159
Group A *Streptococcus* tests,
errors in, 112
Guaiac blood tests, errors in, 113

H
Hair, safety and, 171
Hand hygiene
alcohol-based cleansers in,
157
handwashing guidelines in,
157
Hand veins
anchoring of, 35
palpation of, 34
patient positioning and, 31
selection of, 26
Haptoglobin, 186

Heel puncture
in blood smear collection,
135–136
in capillary blood gas
collection, 130–133
in newborn screening,
125–128
patient positioning for, 118
procedure for, 118–122
site warming in, 126, 131
sites for, 115–116
Hematocrit test, 181–182
Hematoma
alerts regarding, 41, 47
as arterial puncture
complication, 155
as venipuncture complication,
68
Hemoconcentration, as
venipuncture complication,
70
Hemoglobin A1c, 181
Hemoglobin electrophoresis,
181
Hemoglobin tests
description of, 181–182
errors in, 112
Hemolysis, as venipuncture
complication, 71–72
Hemorrhage, as arterial
puncture complication, 155
Heparin
as additive, 6, 17
in arterial blood gas syringes,
148, 154
Heparin anti-X$_a$ assay, 182
Hepatitis A, 174
Hepatitis B core antibody test,
182

Hepatitis B surface antibody test, 182

Hepatitis B surface antigen test, 182

Hepatitis B virus
anti–hepatitis B surface antigen test, 174
immunization against, 158
postexposure testing and prophylaxis for, 167

Hepatitis C virus
anti–hepatitis C virus test, 174
postexposure testing and prophylaxis for, 167–168

Herbs
coagulation and, 62
laboratory tests and, 61

Homocysteine test, 182

Homozygated patients, patient identification in, 28

Human chorionic gonadotropin test, 182

Human immunodeficiency virus
anti-HIV test, 174
postexposure testing and prophylaxis for, 167–168

Hypothyroidism, newborn screening for, 125

I

Ice packing, of chilled specimens, 89

IgA, 186

IgG, 186

IgM, 186

Immunizations. See also specific immunizations
CDC recommendations, 158
personal record of, 159

Immunoassay kits, errors in use of, 112

Immunoglobulin tests, 182

Immunoglobulins, 186

Implanted port, blood collection from, 99–101

Infection
as arterial puncture complication, 155
as venipuncture complication, 67

Infection control, 157–166
blood and body fluid cleanup in, 166
blood and body fluid exposure evaluation in, 167–168
hand hygiene in, 157
immunizations in, 158–159
isolation precautions in, 162–164
patient contact limited in, 158
personal protection equipment in, 159–162
sharps precautions in, 166–167
summary of guidelines in, 168
in unfixed slide handling, 138

Inspection of equipment, 23

Insulin test, 182

International normalized ratio, 182

In-vein retraction device needle, 2

Inversion, of blood collection tubes, 40, 47, 54

Iodine, for blood culture collection, 81

Iron tests, 183

Iron-binding capacity, 183
Isolation precautions
  classification of, 162–164
  phlebotomy procedure and,
    164–165
  protective/reverse, 165
Isopropyl alcohol
  in arterial puncture
    procedure, 146
  in blood collection, 22
i-STAT profiles, errors in, 112

J
Jewelry, safety and, 171

L
Labeling of collection tubes, 6,
  41, 47
Laboratory tests, 173–189. See
  also specific tests
  diurnal variation and, 75
  hemolysis and, 71
  overview of common,
    173–189
  pre-examination variables
    and, 56–60
Lactate dehydrogenase test,
  183
Lactic acid tests
  overview of, 183
  specimen chilling
    recommended after, 154
  venous stasis alert regarding,
    70
Latex allergy
  alerts regarding, 31, 159
  patients asked about, 36, 49,
    118, 135
Lead test, 183

Leg and foot veins,
  venipuncture alerts regarding,
    27
Legal specimens, handling of,
  91–93
Lidocaine, for arterial puncture,
  146
Lifting technique, 171
Light-sensitive specimens,
  handling of, 89–90
Lipase test, 183
Lipoprotein tests, 184
Lithium heparin, in arterial
  blood gas syringes, 148
Lithium test, 184
Local anesthetic, in arterial
  puncture procedure, 146–147
Luer-Lok tip, in syringe system,
  20

M
Magnesium test, 184
Masks
  donning of, 161
  purpose of, 159
  removal of, 162
Measles, mumps, rubella
  immunization, 158
Medications
  glucose tolerance tests
    affected by, 77
  laboratory tests affected by,
    60–61
Microcollection containers, for
  dermal puncture procedures,
    117, 121
Microhematocrit tubes, in
  dermal puncture procedures,
    121

Midstream clean-catch urine specimens
  for cultures, 102
  gender-specific procedures for, 102–103
Modified Allen test, 143–145
Mononucleosis screen, 184
Myocardial infarction panel, 184
Myoglobin test, 184

N

N95 respirators, 159
Needle(s)
  in evacuated tube system, 1–2
  indication for, 65
  punctures caused by, 166–167
  safety alerts regarding, 1–2, 5
  safety features and devices of, 2–3
  safety procedures for, 2
  standard sizes of, 1
  in syringe system, 20
  in venipuncture procedure, 25
Needle holders, 4
Nerve injury
  as arterial puncture complication, 155
  as venipuncture complication, 67–68
Newborn bilirubin testing, ultraviolet light and, 119
Newborn screening
  equipment for, 125
  galactosemia, 125
  heel puncture sites for, 115
  hypothyroidism, 125
  phenylketonuria, 125
  procedure for, 125–128

Nonfasting state, as laboratory test variable, 58

O

Occult blood tests, errors in, 113
Occupational Safety and Health Administration, on needle safety devices, 3
Oral contraceptives, laboratory tests and, 61
Oral glucose tolerance tests, 76–80
Order of draw
  in dermal puncture procedures, 123
  in venipuncture recommended, 15
Osmolality test, 184
Oxalate, as additive, 6
Oxygen content and saturation tests, 140

P

Palpation of veins, in venipuncture, 34, 37, 44, 50
Parathyroid hormone test, 184
Partial pressure of carbon dioxide and oxygen tests, 140–141
Partial thromboplastin time, 185
Partially filled tubes, 73
PASS, in fire protocol, 171
Paternity tests, DNA sampling for, 92
Patient assessment, for arterial puncture, 141
Patient contact, conditions limiting, 158

Patient identification
  alerts regarding, 28, 36, 43, 49
  for capillary blood gas collection, 130
  in dermal puncture procedure, 118
  in newborn screening, 125
  for point of care testing, 110
  for venipuncture, 28
Patient instructions, for midstream clean-catch urine specimens, 102-103
Patient positioning
  alerts regarding, 29, 36, 43, 49
  for dermal puncture procedure, 118
  for venipuncture, 29, 36, 44, 50
Patient refusal, as venipuncture complication, 66
Patient-related complications, of venipuncture, 65-67
Peak levels, in therapeutic drug monitoring, 76
Pediatric patients
  bandages contraindicated in, 128, 133
  capillary blood gas collection in, 130-133
  dermal puncture sites for, 115-116
  newborn screening in, 125-128
  winged blood collection sets in, 21-22

Personal protective equipment
  donning of, 161-162
  in infection control, 159-162
  in isolation precautions, 162-164
  list of, 159
  removal of, 161-162
Petechiae, as venipuncture complication, 66-67
pH test, 141, 185
Phenobarbital test, 187
Phenylketonuria, newborn screening for, 125
Phenytoin test, 187
Phlebotomy procedures. See Arterial puncture; Dermal puncture
Phosphorus test, 185
Physical precautions, 171
Plasminogen test, 185
Platelet aggregation test, 185
Platelet count, 185
Point of care meter errors, 113
Point of care testing, 110-113
  common errors in, 111-113
  dermal puncture in, 110
  error prevention in, 110-111
Polymer barrier gel, as additive, 7
Porphyrin test, 185
Postexposure protocols, for blood and body fluid, 167-168
Posture, as laboratory test variable, 59
Potassium oxalate, 18
Potassium test, 185

Povidone iodine, for blood culture collection, 81
Pre-examination variables, laboratory tests and, 56–60
Pregnancy
  avoidance of radiation in, 170
  errors in tests for, 113
  as laboratory test variable, 59
Preservatives, as additives, 6
Pretest preparation, in venipuncture procedure, 36, 43, 49
Prostate-specific antigen test, 186
Prostatic acid phosphatase, 186
Protective isolation procedures, 165
Protein electrophoresis, 186
Protein test, 186
Prothrombin time test
  chilling contraindicated for specimens for, 89
  description of, 91, 186

Q

Quality control
  of equipment, 23
  for point-of-care testing, 111
Quantitative protein assay, 186

R

RACE, in fire protocol, 171
Radial artery puncture, 148–153
  anatomic site of, 142
  equipment for, 148
  modified Allen test before, 143–145
  as preferred arterial site, 142

pressure application after, 151–152
procedure for, 148–153
syringe size in, 148
weak pulse after, 153
Radiation
  precautions regarding, 169–170
  symbol designating, 170
Random urine specimens, 102
Rapid immunological group A strep test, throat specimen collection for, 105–109
Rapid plasma reagin test, 186
Red blood cell count, 186
Reporting, of blood and body fluid exposure, 167
Requisition forms
  for arterial puncture, 141, 149
  for blood collection from implanted port, 99
  for blood smear collection, 135
  for capillary blood gas collection, 130
  for dermal puncture, 118
  for newborn screening, 125
  for venipuncture, 25, 28, 36, 43, 49
Respirators, in personal protective equipment, 159
Result interpretation, for point of care testing, 111
Reticulocyte count, 91, 186
Reverse isolation procedures, 165
Rheumatoid factor test, 180
Rubella titer, 187

S

Safety, 157–172
    chart for equipment location in, 172
    chemical precautions in, 169
    electrical precautions in, 170–171
    fire and explosion precautions in, 171
    infection control in, 157–166
    needle devices and features promoting, 2–3
    physical precautions in, 171
    radiation precautions in, 169–170
    sharps precautions in, 166–167
Safety Data Sheet, chemical indications for, 169
Safety shield, 2
Salicylate test, 187
Scarred skin, venipuncture avoided in, 27
Screening, newborn. *See* Newborn screening
Seizures, as venipuncture complication, 66–67
Serum separator tubes, 73
Sharps. *See also* Needle(s)
    disposal containers for, 5
    disposal procedure for, 41
    precautions for, 166–167
Shock, electrical, 171
Sickle cell screening, 187
Silica, as additive, 7
Smoking, as laboratory test variable, 59–60
Sodium citrate, 18

Sodium fluoride, as additive, 7, 19
Sodium heparin, in arterial blood gas syringes, 148
Sodium polyanethol sulfonate
    as additive, 6
    in blood culture bottles, 80–81
Special procedures, 75–114
Special specimen handling, 88 94
Specimen
    coagulation, 90
    collection of, in error prevention, 110–111
    preparation of, in venipuncture procedure, 41, 48
    rejection of, 73–74
    storage of, 90–91
Spore-forming bacteria, alcohol-based cleansers and, 157
Standing position, alerts against, 29, 49
Sterile technique. *See* Aseptic technique
Storage
    of specimen, 90–91
    of testing supplies for point of care testing, 110
Strep testing, throat specimen collection for, 105–109
Stress, as laboratory test variable, 60
Suprapubic aspirations, in urine collection, 102
Syncope, as venipuncture complication, 65–66

Syringe system
  for central venous catheter
    collection, 95
  components of, 20, 43
  venipuncture using, 43–48

T

T-cell count, 187
Technical venipuncture
  complications
  errors affecting patients as,
    67–69
  errors affecting specimens as,
    70–74
  failure to obtain blood as,
    63–65
Tegretol (carbamazepine),
  177
Temperature-sensitive
  specimens, handling of,
  88–90
Testosterone test, 187
Tests. See specific test
Tetanus immunization, 158
Theophylline test, 187
Therapeutic drug monitoring,
  medications in, 75–76
Throat culture
  equipment for, 106
  specimen collection for,
    105–109
Thrombin, as additive, 7
Thrombus formation, as
  arterial puncture
  complication, 156
Thumb, vein palpation
  contraindicated with, 34
Thyroid-stimulating hormone,
  187

Timed specimens
  diurnal variation and, 75
  reasons for, 75
  therapeutic drug monitoring
    and, 75–76
  24-hour urine specimen
    collection, 104
Tissue destruction, as arterial
  puncture complication, 156
Total protein test, 187
Tourniquets
  alerts regarding, 31, 34, 37,
    44, 50
  equipment for, 31–32
  in venipuncture procedure,
    31–34, 37, 44, 50
Toxicology profiles, errors in,
  113
Training, for central venous
  catheter collection, 94
Transmission-based isolation
  precautions, 162–164
Triglyceride test, 188
Troponin tests, 188
Trough drug levels, in
  therapeutic drug monitoring,
  76
Tube system, evacuated,
  1–4
Tuberculosis skin test,
  158
Type and screen, 188

U

Ulnar artery testing, before
  radial artery puncture,
  143–145
Ultraviolet light, in newborn
  bilirubin tests, 119

Uric acid test, 188
Urinalysis, errors in, 113
Urine tests
  for drugs, 92–93
  errors in, 113
  midstream clean-catch
    collection for, 102–103
  pregnancy, 113
  specimen collection types for,
    102–105
  timed (24-hour) collection for,
    104

V

Vacuette collection tubes, 12–14
Valproic acid test, 187–188
Varicella immunization, 158
Vascular access devices, 101
Vasovagal reaction, as arterial
  puncture complication, 156
Veins
  anchoring of, 35, 38, 45, 51
  arm and hand, 26
  enhancement methods for, 27
  palpation of, 34, 37, 44, 50
  for venipuncture, 26–27. See
    also Venipuncture
Venereal Disease Research
  Laboratory test, 188
Venipuncture, 25–55
  anchoring of veins in, 35, 38,
    45, 51
  arm and hand veins for, 26
  bandage in, 41–42, 48
  complications of, 56–74. See
    also Complications; specific
    complication
  evacuated tube systems,
    35–42

for glucose tolerance tests, 78
  hematoma alerts in, 41, 47
  in isolation, 164–165
  labeling of tubes in, 6, 41, 47
  needles for, 1–2. See also
    Needle(s)
  palpation of veins in, 34, 37,
    44, 50
  patient identification for, 28
  patient positioning for, 29–31,
    36, 44, 50
  procedure checklist for, 25
  sites to avoid in, 27
  specimen preparation in, 41,
    48
  syringe systems, 43–48
  tourniquets in, 31–34, 37, 44,
    50
  vein enhancement for, 27
  winged blood collection sets,
    49–55
Venous blood, arterial blood
  gas test errors from, 155
Viral infections, isolation
  precautions for, 162–164
Vitamins
  coagulation and, 62
  tests for, 188–189
Vomiting, in glucose tolerance
  tests, 78

W

Warming of heel puncture
  site
  for capillary blood gas
    collection, 131
  in newborn screening, 126
Weak pulse, after arterial
  puncture, 153

Wedge arm support, for
  venipuncture, 31
Western blot test, 189
White blood cell count, 189
Winged blood collection sets
  for blood culture, 81
  components of, 21–22, 49

uses of, 21–22
venipuncture using, 49–55
Wrist, venipuncture avoided in,
  27

Z
Zinc tests, 189

document GP42-A6. Clinical and Laboratory Standards Institute, Wayne, PA, 2008.

CLSI. Procedures for the Handling and Processing of Blood Specimens for Common Laboratory Tests. Approved Guideline, ed. 4. CLSI document GP44-A4. Clinical and Laboratory Standards Institute, Wayne, PA, 2012.

CLSI. Tubes and Additives for Venous and Capillary Blood Specimen Collection, ed. 6. Approved Standard GP39-A6. Clinical and Laboratory Standards Institute, Wayne, PA, 2010.

Methodist Hospital Nursing Service Policy and Procedure Manual: Blood Specimen Collection From Vascular Access Device. Methodist Hospital, Omaha, NE, 2014.

Strasinger S. K., & Di Lorenzo, M. S. The Phlebotomy Textbook, 4th ed. Philadelphia: F.A. Davis, 2019.

Vacuette Blood Collection System—Handling Recommendations. Available at: www.gbo.com/preanalytics.

Index

A

Accidental arterial puncture, as venipuncture complication, 69

Acetaminophen, laboratory tests and, 60

Acid, post-contact protocol for, 169

Acid citrate dextrose
as additive, 6
for DNA specimens, 92

Acid phosphatase test, 173

Activated partial thromboplastin time, 90, 185

Additives in blood collection tubes. *See also specific additives*
overview of, 6–14
tests affected by, 17–19

Adrenocorticotropic hormone test, 173

Adulteration prevention in urine drug testing, 92–93

Age, as laboratory test variable, 56

Air bubbles, arterial blood gas test errors from, 154

Airborne transmission, infection control precautions in, 162

Alanine aminotransferase test, 173

Albumin test, 173

Alcohol
for blood culture equipment cleansing, 81, 84
in central venous catheter collection, 96

Alcohol consumption
glucose tolerance tests affected by, 76–77
as laboratory test variable, 56

Alcohol-based cleansers, for hand hygiene, 157

Aldosterone test, 173

Alkaline phosphatase test, 173

Alpha-fetoprotein test, 173

Altitude, as laboratory test variable, 56

Aluminum foil, for light-sensitive specimens, 90

Aluminum test, 173

Amber-colored containers, for light-sensitive specimens, 90

Ammonia test, 174

Amylase test, 174

Anchoring of veins, in venipuncture, 35, 38, 45, 51

Angiotensin-converting enzyme test, 174

Antibiotics
assays of, 174
therapeutic monitoring of, 75–76

Antibody ID/screen, 174

Anticoagulants
as additives, 6–7
in arterial blood gas syringes, 148
for blood culture, 81
tube inversion with, 40, 47, 54

Newborn Screening

Newborn screening tests are performed on blood collected by dermal puncture between 24 and 72 hours after birth. Specimens should be collected separately, after prewarming and puncturing a second site when additional blood tests are requested. Each state has its own laws requiring specific test screening of newborns; however, all states test for phenylketonuria, congenital hypothyroidism, and galactosemia.

Equipment

- Newborn screening filter paper form
- Gloves
- 70% isopropyl alcohol pads
- Heel puncture device
- 2-inch × 2-inch gauze
- Warming device
- Sharps disposal container
- Indelible pen

Procedure

1. Obtain and examine the requisition form. Check for completeness, date and time of collection, and priority.
2. Greet the patient's parents, and explain the procedure.
3. Identify the patient using two identifiers. Ask a parent or guardian to identify an infant or a child. Compare the ID band with the requisition form.

ALERT: The ID band must be **on** an infant.

4. Assemble the proper equipment.
5. Sanitize your hands using the proper technique.
6. Apply gloves, and put on a gown if required by the nursery.
7. Position the patient.

DERMAL
PUNCT

DERMAL PUNCT

8. For optimal blood flow, warm the area to be punctured either by:
   - Placing a towel that has been moistened with warm water (42°C) on the site (requires you to dry the site before puncture), or
   - Activating a commercial warmer and covering the site for 3 to 5 minutes.
9. Cleanse the site with 70% isopropyl alcohol, and allow it to air-dry.
10. Prepare the lancet by removing the lancet locking device.
11. Grasp the heel with your nondominant hand. Encircle the heel with your index finger around the arch, your thumb around the bottom, and your other fingers around the top of the foot.
12. Place the lancet firmly on the fleshy medial or lateral plantar surface area of the heel perpendicular to the heelprint.
13. Depress the lancet trigger.
14. Discard the lancet in an approved sharps disposal container.

💢 **ALERT:** Failure to place the puncture device firmly on the skin is the primary cause of insufficient blood flow.

15. Gently squeeze the heel.
16. Wipe away the first drop of blood because it may contain alcohol residue and tissue fluid.
17. Touch the filter paper to a large drop of blood.

💢 **ALERT:** Do not press the paper against the heel.

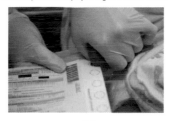

18. With **one drop** of blood, evenly fill the circle on one side of the filter paper, allowing the blood to soak through the preprinted circle on the filter paper. Examine both sides of the paper to confirm that the blood has uniformly penetrated and saturated through the paper.

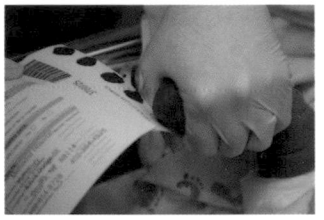

🖐 **ALERT:** Avoid touching or smearing the blood on the filter paper.

🖐 **ALERT:** Uneven or incomplete saturation of filter paper circles will yield an unacceptable specimen for testing.

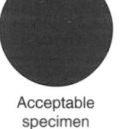

Acceptable specimen

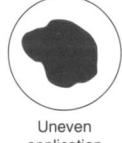

Uneven application of blood

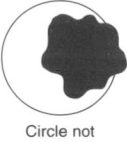

Circle not completely filled

19. Fill all required circles correctly.

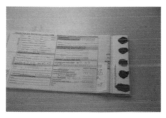

20. Place gauze on the site, elevate the foot, and apply pressure until the bleeding stops.
21. Check the site for bleeding.

🖐 **ALERT:** Do not place an adhesive bandage on children younger than age 2 years.

22. Dispose of used supplies.
23. Remove all collection equipment from the area.
24. Remove your gloves.
25. Sanitize your hands.
26. Complete the patient log sheet.
27. Place the filter paper in a suspended horizontal position on an open surface for 3 hours at ambient temperature and away from direct sunlight to allow it to dry.

🖐 **ALERT:** Do not stack multiple filter papers when drying.

28. After the blood dries, label the specimen and place it in the special envelope.

🖐 **ALERT:** Allow the blood spots to thoroughly dry before folding the attached flap over the spots.

29. Deliver the specimen to the laboratory for mailing to the reference testing agency.

_____
_____
_____
_____
_____
_____
_____
_____
_____
_____
_____
_____
_____
_____
_____
_____
_____
_____
_____
_____
_____

Newborn Screening Notes

Capillary Blood Gas Collection by Heel Puncture

Because deep arterial punctures are not recommended for newborns and young children, blood gas analysis is performed on capillary blood collected by heel puncture.

Equipment

- Requisition form
- Gloves
- 70% isopropyl alcohol pads
- Heel puncture device
- Heparinized capillary tubes with caps
- Metal stirrer "flea"
- Round magnet
- Warming device
- 2-inch × 2-inch gauze
- Sharps disposal container
- Indelible pen
- Ice slurry, if needed

Procedure

1. Obtain and examine the requisition form. Check for completeness, date and time of collection, and priority.
2. Greet the patient and his or her parents, and explain the procedure.
3. Identify the patient using two identifiers. Ask a parent or guardian to identify an infant or a child. Also, match the ID band with the requisition form.

🖑 ALERT: The ID band must be **on** an infant.

4. Select the proper equipment.
5. Sanitize your hands using the proper technique.
6. Apply gloves, and put on a gown if required by the nursery.
7. Position the patient.
8. For optimal blood flow, warm the area to be punctured either by:
   - Placing a towel that has been moistened with warm water (42°C) on the site (requires you to dry the site before puncture), or

130

- Activating a commercial warmer and covering the site for 3 to 5 minutes.
9. Cleanse the site with 70% isopropyl alcohol, and allow it to air-dry.
10. Prepare the lancet by removing the lancet locking device.

11. Grasp the heel with your nondominant hand. Wrap your index finger around the arch, your thumb around the bottom, and your other fingers around the top of the foot.
12. Place the lancet firmly on the fleshy medial or lateral plantar surface area of the heel perpendicular to the heelprint.
13. Depress the lancet trigger.
14. Discard the lancet in an approved sharps disposal container.

✋ **ALERT:** Failure to place the puncture device firmly on the skin is the primary cause of insufficient blood flow.

15. Gently squeeze the finger or heel.
16. Wipe away the first drop of blood because it may contain alcohol residue and tissue fluid.
17. Hold the capillary tube horizontal to the drop of blood and fill the capillary tube in less than 30 seconds to avoid exposing the blood to air.

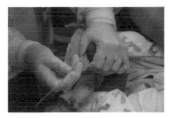

18. Completely fill the tube without any air spaces. Place the magnetic "flea" in the capillary tube.

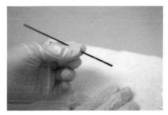

19. Immediately seal both ends of the capillary tube.

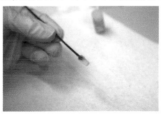

20. Mix the specimen in the heparin-coated tube by moving the magnet up and down the tube several times. The "flea" should move from one end to the other end of the specimens.

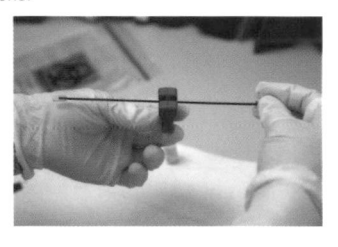

👆 **ALERT:** Avoid creating bubbles in the specimens.

21. Place gauze on the site, and apply pressure until the bleeding stops.
22. Label the tubes.
23. Place the tubes in an ice water slurry if testing is not performed within 15 minutes.
24. Check the site for bleeding.

👆 **ALERT:** Do not place an adhesive bandage on children younger than age 2 years.

25. Dispose of used supplies.
26. Remove all collection equipment from the area.
27. Remove your gloves.
28. Sanitize your hands.
29. Thank the parents if present.
30. Complete the patient log sheet.
31. Promptly deliver the specimens to the laboratory.

Capillary Blood Gas Collection Notes

_____

_____

_____

_____

_____

_____

_____

_____

_____

_____

_____

Preparation of Blood Smears

Blood smears, which can be collected by dermal puncture, are needed for the microscopic examination of blood cells for differential blood cell counts, for special staining procedures, and for nonautomated reticulocyte counts.

Equipment
- Gloves
- 70% isopropyl alcohol pads
- Finger or heel puncture device
- Three plain or frosted glass slides, free of cracked or chipped edges
- 2-inch × 2-inch gauze
- Warming device
- Sharps disposal container
- Pencil
- Bandage

Procedure

1. Obtain and examine the requisition form. Check for completeness, date and time of collection, and priority.
2. Greet the patient, and explain the procedure.
3. Identify the patient using two identifiers.
4. Ask about latex allergies and previous problems with blood collection.
5. Position the patient.
6. Assemble the proper equipment.
7. Sanitize your hands using the proper technique.
8. Apply gloves.
9. Select the puncture site.
10. For optimal blood flow, warm the area to be punctured either by:
    - Placing a towel that has been moistened with warm water (42°C) on the site, or
    - Activating a commercial warmer and covering the site for 3 to 5 minutes.
11. Cleanse the site with 70% isopropyl alcohol, and allow it to air-dry.
12. Prepare the lancet by removing the lancet locking device.
13. Grasp and position the area to be punctured:
    - **For a heelstick,** grasp the heel with your index finger around the arch, your thumb around the bottom, and your other fingers around the top of the foot.
    - **For a fingerstick,** hold the finger between your nondominant thumb and index finger, with the palmar surface facing up and the finger pointing downward.
14. Place the lancet firmly on the fleshy area of the finger or heel perpendicular to the fingerprint or heelprint.
15. Depress the lancet trigger.
16. Discard the lancet in an approved sharps disposal container.

ALERT: Failure to place the puncture device firmly on the skin is the primary cause of insufficient blood flow.

17. Gently squeeze the finger or heel.
18. Wipe away the first drop of blood.
19. Place the second drop of blood in the center of a glass slide approximately $\frac{1}{2}$ inch to 1 inch from the end or just below the frosted end by lightly touching the drop with the slide. The drop should be 1 to 2 mm in diameter.

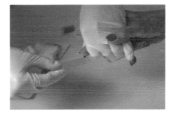

20. Place a second slide (spreader slide) with a clean, smooth edge in front of the drop at a 30- to 40-degree angle inclined over the blood.

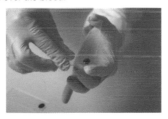

DERMAL PUNCT

21. Draw the spreader slide back to the edge of the drop of blood, allowing the blood to spread across the end.

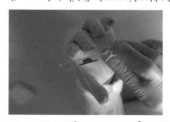

22. When the blood is evenly distributed across the spreader slide, lightly push the spreader slide forward with a continuous movement all the way past the end of the smear.
   - Maintain the 30- to 40-degree angle.
   - Do not apply pressure to the spreader slide.
   - Cover one-half to two-thirds of the slide, without ridges or holes and with a feathered edge without streaks.

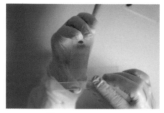

23. Place the slide in an area where it can dry undisturbed.

💧 **ALERT:** Do not blow on a slide to dry it because doing so can cause red blood cell distortion.

24. Repeat the procedure for the second smear using the clean side of the spreader slide.
25. Place gauze on the site, and apply pressure until the bleeding stops.
26. Label the frosted ends by writing the patient's information on the frosted area with a pencil. Attach preprinted labels to the thick end of smear slides that do not have frosted ends.

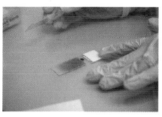

Place the slides in a biohazard transport container. Place the contaminated spreader slides in the sharps container.

27. Remove your gloves.
28. Sanitize your hands.
29. Promptly deliver the slides to the laboratory.

🖐 **ALERT.** Wear gloves when handling unfixed slides because they are capable of transmitting disease.

Preparation of Blood Smears Notes

_____

_____

_____

_____

_____

_____

_____

_____

_____

_____

_____

_____

_____

_____

_____

_____

_____

_____

_____

_____

DERMAL PUNCT

Arterial Blood Collection

Arterial blood is requested primarily for the evaluation of blood gases (oxygen and carbon dioxide) to evaluate respiratory function.

Arterial Blood Gas Tests		
Test	Description	Normal Value
Base excess or deficit	• Reflects the nonrespiratory part of acid-base balance based on Pco_2, HCO_3^-, and hemoglobin	$(-2) - (+2)$ mEq/L
Bicarbonate (HCO_3^-)	• Evaluates the bicarbonate buffer system of the kidneys that prevents acidosis and alkalosis	20–29 mEq/L
Oxygen content (cto_2)	• Measures the amount of oxygen in the blood	15–22 mL/100 mL of blood
Oxygen saturation (O_2Sat)	• Measures how much of the hemoglobin in the red blood cells is carrying oxygen	95%–100%
Partial pressure of carbon dioxide (Pco_2)	• Measures the pressure of carbon dioxide dissolved in the blood • Indicates how well carbon dioxide moves out of the lungs • Helps to evaluate lung function	35–45 mm Hg

Continued

Arterial Blood Gas Tests—cont'd

Test	Description	Normal Value
Partial pressure of oxygen (PO_2)	• Measures the pressure of oxygen dissolved in the blood • Indicates how well oxygen moves from the lungs into the blood • Helps to evaluate if ventilation is adequate	75–100 mm mercury (Hg)
pH	• Measures the acidity or alkalinity of the blood • Indicates acidosis or alkalosis	7.35–7.45

Patient Assessment

Patient information that must be recorded on the patient test requisition form includes:

■ Time of collection
■ Patient's temperature
■ Patient's respiratory rate
■ Method of ventilation
■ Amount of oxygen the patient is receiving
■ Patient activity
■ Collection site and method

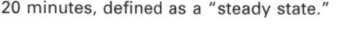 **ALERT:** Confirm that the patient has been receiving the specified amount of oxygen and has refrained from exercise for at least 20 minutes, defined as a "steady state."

ARTERIAL PUNCT

Site Selection

Artery Selection Criteria
- Large enough to accept a 25-gauge needle
- Located near the skin's surface
- Located in an area where injury to surrounding tissues will not be critical
- Located in an area where other arteries are present to supply blood (collateral circulation) in case the punctured artery is damaged

ARTERIAL PUNCTURE SITES

- Radial: Located on the thumb side of the wrist, artery of choice

👋 **ALERT:** The radial artery is preferred for arterial puncture.

- Brachial: Located in the antecubital fossa near the basilic vein
- Femoral: Located near the groin

👋 **ALERT:** The femoral artery should be used for arterial puncture only by physicians and specially trained personnel.

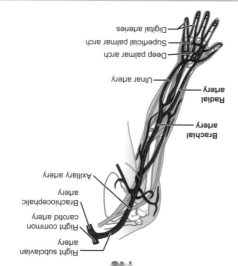

Digital arteries
Superficial palmar arch
Deep palmar arch
Ulnar artery
Radial artery
Radial artery
Brachial artery
Axillary artery
Brachiocephalic artery
Right common carotid artery
Right subclavian artery

Modified Allen Test

Procedure

1. Extend the patient's wrist over a rolled towel.
2. Ask the patient to form a tight fist.
3. Locate the pulses of the radial and ulnar arteries on the palmar surface of the wrist by palpating with the middle and index fingers—not the thumb, which has a pulse.
4. Compress both arteries at the same time.

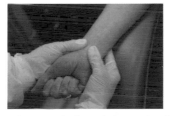

5. Have the patient open the fist and observe that the palm has become pale (blanched).

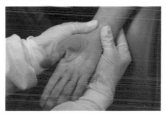

6. Release pressure on the ulnar artery only and watch to see that color returns to the palm. This should occur within 15 seconds if the ulnar artery is functioning.

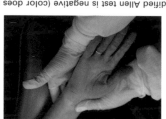

7. If the modified Allen test is negative (color does not appear), do not use the radial artery for specimen collection.

8. If the modified Allen test is positive (color appears), proceed by palpating the radial artery to determine its depth, direction, and size.

9. Record the results on the requisition form.

Notes

_____

_____

_____

_____

_____

_____

_____

_____

_____

_____

_____

_____

Site Preparation

- If needed, a local anesthetic should be administered prior to beginning the actual site-cleansing procedure.
- Because the risk of infection is higher in arterial punctures than in venipunctures, cleanliness of the site is very important. The puncture site should be cleaned with 70% isopropyl alcohol and allowed to air-dry.
- The gloved palpating fingers should be cleansed in the same manner.

PREPARING AND ADMINISTRATING THE LOCAL ANESTHETIC

Equipment
- Gloves
- 25- or 26-gauge needle
- 1-mL syringe
- 1% lidocaine without epinephrine
- 70% isopropyl alcohol pad
- Sharps disposal container

Procedure
1. Obtain the requisition form and check it for completeness.
2. Greet and identify the patient using two identifiers.
3. Explain the procedure, reassure the patient, and obtain consent.
4. Ask about allergies to the anesthetic.
5. Sanitize your hands.
6. Put on gloves.
7. Attach the needle to the syringe.
8. Cleanse the vial top with isopropyl alcohol.
9. Insert the needle through the vial top and withdraw 0.5 mL of anesthetic solution (lidocaine).
10. Recap the needle and place it horizontally on the table.
11. Locate the puncture site.
12. Cleanse the puncture site with alcohol.
13. Allow it to air-dry.

14. Using your nondominant hand, raise the intradermal layer of the patient's skin slightly above the artery.
15. Hold the needle at about a 10-degree angle, and puncture the raised skin subcutaneously.
16. Slightly pull back on the syringe plunger before injecting the lidocaine to be sure that blood does not appear, indicating puncture of a blood vessel.
17. Slowly inject the anesthetic, forming a raised wheal.
18. Remove the needle.
19. Allow 2 to 3 minutes for the anesthetic to take effect.
20. Proceed with the arterial puncture procedure when the patient has relaxed.
21. Document administration of the anesthetic on the requisition form.

Notes

_____

_____

_____

_____

_____

_____

_____

_____

_____

_____

_____

_____

_____

_____

ARTERIAL
PUNCT

Arterial Puncture Procedure

RADIAL ARTERY PUNCTURE PROCEDURE

Equipment
■ Requisition Gloves form
■ 70% Alcohol pads
■ Heparinized blood gas syringe
■ Needle with safety device

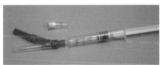

👆 **ALERT:** Plastic blood gas syringes that are precoated with sodium or lithium heparin and specifically designed for ABG specimens are recommended. If electrolytes are also ordered, use a lithium-coated (not sodium-coated) syringe.

👆 **ALERT:** Syringes should be no larger than the volume needed for the requested tests.

■ Luer cap
■ Gauze pads
■ Self-adhesive pressure bandage
■ Ice slurry, if necessary
■ Indelible pen
■ Sharps disposal container
■ Biohazard bag

Procedure

1. Obtain and examine the requisition form. Check for completeness.
2. Greet the patient. Have the patient state his or her first and last names, spell the last name, and state the date of birth.
3. Explain the procedure, reassure the patient, and obtain consent.
4. Ask about allergies.
5. Obtain oxygen therapy information and ensure that the patient is in a steady state.
6. Record required information.
7. Sanitize your hands.
8. Put on gloves.
9. Organize the equipment.
10. Set the syringe plunger to the correct fill level if applicable.
11. Support and hyperextend the patient's wrist.

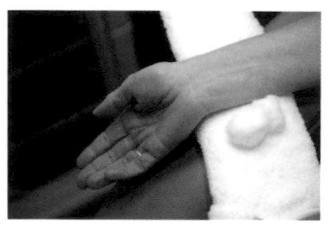

12. Perform the modified Allen test.
13. Locate and palpate the radial artery.

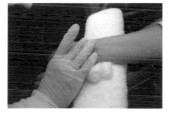

14. Cleanse the site and the palpating finger with alcohol.
15. Uncap and inspect the needle.
16. Place a clean, gloved, nondominant finger over the arterial puncture site.

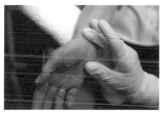

17. Insert the needle, bevel up, at a 30- to 45-degree angle, 10 to 15 mm below the palpating finger. Stop when a flash of blood appears.

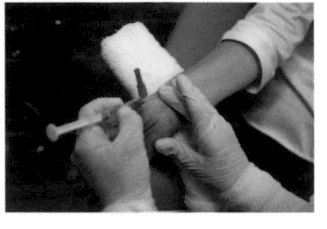

✋ **ALERT:** Avoid probing to find the artery because doing so can cause pain, a hematoma, or thrombus formation.

18. Allow the syringe to fill to the designated level.
19. Place clean, folded gauze over the site; remove the needle; and apply pressure.

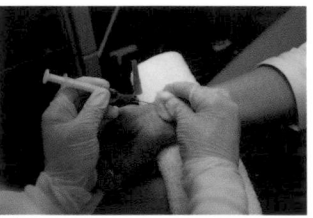

20. Activate the safety shield while maintaining pressure on the site.

✋ **ALERT:** The blood collector, not the patient, must apply firm pressure for a minimum of 3 minutes or until bleeding has completely stopped.

ARTERIAL
PUNCT

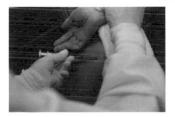

21. Remove the needle while maintaining pressure.

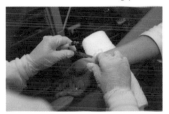

22. Discard the needle in the sharps disposal container.
23. Expel air bubbles, apply a Luer cap device, and mix the syringe thoroughly by rotating while retaining pressure.

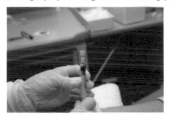

24. If the test is not going to be performed within 30 minutes, place the specimen, collected in a glass syringe, in an ice slurry.
25. Check the puncture site for bleeding after 3 to 5 minutes. Maintain pressure if bleeding has not stopped.
26. Label the specimen after bleeding has stopped.
27. Reexamine the puncture site.
28. Check for a radial pulse.

👆 ALERT: Notify a supervisor immediately if the pulse is weak or absent.

29. Apply a pressure bandage if the site and pulse are normal.
30. Dispose of contaminated materials.
31. Remove gloves.
32. Sanitize your hands.
33. Thank the patient.
34. Immediately deliver specimen to the laboratory.

Notes

_____

_____

_____

_____

_____

_____

_____

_____

_____

_____

_____

_____

ARTERIAL
PUNCT

Specimen Integrity

- Current CLSI recommendations state that specimens that will be analyzed within 30 minutes should be collected in plastic syringes and not placed in an ice bath.
- The exception to this is when lactate (lactic acid) tests have been ordered with the ABG; these specimens should be immediately iced.
- Specimens that cannot be analyzed within 30 minutes should be collected in glass syringes and placed in ice and water.

💧 **ALERT:** ABG test results can be noticeably affected by improper specimen collection and handling.

Effects of Technical Errors on ABG Results	
Technical Error	**Effect**
Air bubbles present	Atmospheric oxygen that has entered the specimen leads to inaccurate test results.
Too much heparin	pH is lowered.
Too little heparin or inadequate mixing	The presence of clots can interfere with the analyzer and lead to erroneous results.

Continued

Effects of Technical Errors on ABG Results—cont'd

Technical Error	Effect
Venous rather than arterial specimen	PO_2 is falsely decreased. PCO_2 is falsely increased.
Delayed analysis	White blood cells and platelets in the specimen continue their metabolism, utilizing oxygen and producing carbon dioxide.

👋 **ALERT:** Blood that does not pulse into the syringe and appears dark rather than bright red may be venous blood and should not be used.

Arterial Puncture Complications

Complication	Cause	Prevention
Hematoma	Arterial blood entering the tissue	Application of pressure until bleeding stops
Hemorrhage	Coagulation disorders and thrombolytic therapy	Increased pressure Use of smaller-gauge needle
Infection	Failure to adequately cleanse the site	Proper cleansing Use of sterile technique
Nerve damage	Deep punctures or improper redirection of the needle	Avoidance of deep sites Additional training for deep sites

Continued

Arterial Puncture Complications—cont'd

Complication	Cause	Prevention
Tissue destruction or gangrene	Arteriospasm (needle penetrates the artery muscle, causing an involuntary contraction of the artery)	Evaluation of collateral circulation
Thrombus formation	Irritation to the inner wall of the artery that obstructs blood flow	Evaluation of collateral circulation
Vasovagal reaction	Apprehension or pain	Reassurance to keep the patient calm Local anesthetic

Notes

_____

_____

_____

_____

_____

_____

_____

_____

_____

Infection Control

Hand Hygiene

CDC Hand Washing Guidelines

- Wet hands with warm water.
- Apply soap.
- Rub hands together to form a lather, create friction, and loosen debris.
- Thoroughly clean hands for at least 20 seconds; be sure to clean between the fingers, under the fingernails, under rings, and around the thumbs and wrists.
- Rinse hands in a downward position to prevent recontamination.
- Obtain a paper towel from the dispenser.
- Dry hands with the paper towel.
- Turn off faucets using a clean paper towel to prevent recontamination.

✋ ALERT: The Centers for Disease Control and Prevention (CDC) recommends against wearing artificial nails in patient settings. Observe your facility's protocol.

Use of Alcohol-Based Cleansers

Alcohol-based cleansers can be used when hands are not visibly contaminated.

- Apply the cleanser to the palm of one hand.
- Rub hands together and over the entire cleansing area, including between the fingers and thumbs.
- Continue rubbing until the alcohol dries.

✋ ALERT: Alcohol-based cleansers are not recommended after contact with spore-forming bacteria, including *Clostridium difficile* and *Bacillus* species, which have become a major source of hospital-associated infections (HAIs).

Immunizations

CDC Immunization Recommendations for Blood Collectors

- Hepatitis B virus (HBV)
  - Completion of three-shot immunization protocol
  - Positive antibody titer
- Measles, mumps, and rubella (MMR)
  - Current positive antibody titer
- Varicella (chickenpox)
  - Current positive antibody titer
- Tetanus
  - Immunization within the past 10 years
- Annual tuberculosis skin test (TST-PPD)
  - Initial testing using the TB two-step procedure (initial and retest 1–3 weeks later)
  - Negative test result on PPD
  - Chest radiograph after positive test result

💧 **ALERT:** In some people, a previous bacille Calmette-Guerin (BCG) vaccine may cause a false positive TST. Those individuals may need to have blood testing performed instead of the TST.

CONDITIONS THAT CAN LIMIT PATIENT CONTACT

- Chickenpox
- Conjunctivitis
- Diarrheal disorders
- Hepatitis A virus
- Herpes zoster/shingles
- Impetigo
- Influenza
- Mumps
- Pediculosis/lice
- Pertussis/whooping cough
- Respiratory syncytial virus (RSV)
- Rubella
- Scabies
- *Streptococcus* group A/ strep throat
- Tuberculosis (active)

Work status involving patient contact varies with institutional regulations determined by the Employee Health Department and may require physician clearance.

Personal Immunization Information

Vaccine	Date Received	Titer	Notes
HBV			
MMR			
Varicella			
Tetanus			
PPD			

Personal Protective Equipment (PPE)

■ Gloves must be worn at all times when collecting, processing, or testing specimens and must be changed between patients.

👆 **ALERT:** Report any latex allergy symptoms to your supervisor.

👆 **ALERT:** Check for latex allergy warnings in patients' rooms. Use latex-free gloves and tourniquets on patients with warnings.

■ **Gowns** must provide full-body coverage.
■ **Masks** protect against droplet inhalation and mucous membrane exposure to droplets.
■ **Goggles** protect the mucous membranes of the eyes.
■ **N95 respirators** protect against airborne organisms such as *Mycobacterium tuberculosis*. They are individually fitted.

Donning PPE

Step 1. Put on the gown and tie it at the neck and waist.

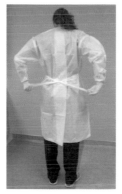

Step 2. Fit the mask to the nose and mouth and then fasten it.

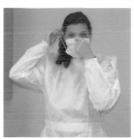

Step 3. Put on goggles and faceshields, if necessary.
Step 4. Pull on gloves over the cuffs of the gown.

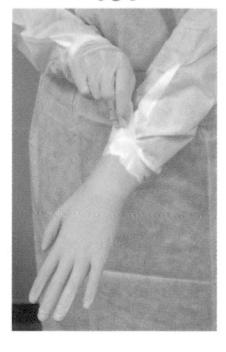

Removing PPE

Remove PPE in the order of most contaminated to least contaminated.

Step 1. Remove and dispose of gloves:

■ Using the other gloved hand, pull off the first glove (starting at the wrist and pulling down) so that the first glove ends up inside out in the still-gloved hand.

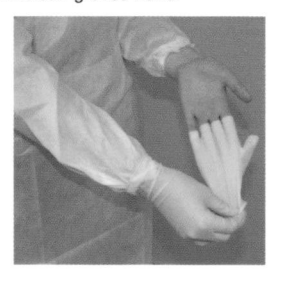

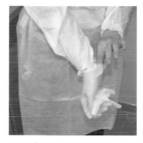

- Slide the ungloved finger inside the glove of the other hand.
- Remove the glove without touching the outside (see previous images).
- Dispose of both gloves.

Step 2. Untie the gown and remove it by touching only the inside of the gown. Dispose of the gown.

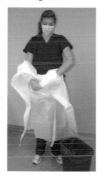

Step 3. Remove the mask touching only the ties or bands. Dispose of the mask.

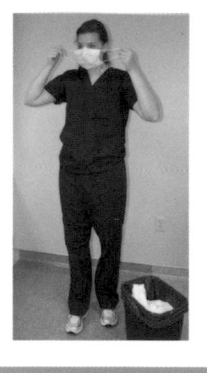

Transmission-Based (Isolation) Precautions

Transmission-Based Precautions Classifications

Type	Possible Conditions	Required Precautions and PPE
Airborne	• Tuberculosis • Measles • Chickenpox • Herpes zoster/shingles • Mumps • Adenovirus	• Standard precautions • Mask or respirator

Continued

SAFETY

Type	Possible Conditions	Required Precautions and PPE
Droplet	• Infection with *Neisseria meningitides* • *Haemophilus* species • Pertussis/whooping cough • Group A *Streptococcus* • Influenza • Rhinovirus • Scarlet fever • Parvovirus B19 • Respiratory syncytial virus • Diphtheria	• Standard precautions • Mask
Contact	• *C. difficile* • Rotavirus • Draining wounds • Antibiotic-resistant infections • Scabies • Impetigo • Herpes simplex virus • Respiratory syncytial virus • Herpes zoster/shingles	• Standard precautions • Gown • Gloves

Performing a Phlebotomy Procedure in Isolation

Before the Procedure

■ Check PPE precaution signs posted on the patient's door to determine the PPE needed to enter the room.

■ Bring only necessary equipment, including extra tubes and supplies to perform a second venipuncture, if necessary.

✋ **ALERT:** Do not bring the phlebotomy tray into the room.

■ Fold open plastic bag or bags and place near or just outside the door.

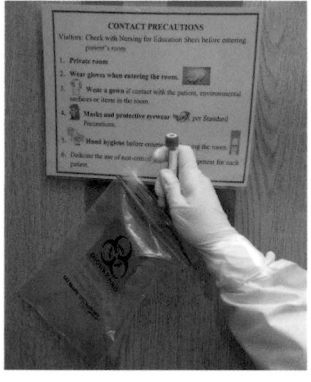

After the Procedure

■ Remove all PPE in the room and leave it in the room.
■ Leave all phlebotomy equipment in the room.
■ Clean the specimen tubes of outside blood and then place them in the plastic bags located near or just outside the door.

👋 **ALERT:** Do not touch the outside of the bags with your gloves or the collection tubes.

Protective/Reverse Isolation Procedures

Patients with compromised immune systems must be protected from routinely encountered organisms carried by the blood collector. Observe the following protective/reverse isolation precautions:

■ Wear sterile PPE.
■ Take only necessary equipment into the room.
■ Remove from the room all equipment that you bring in.
■ Remove PPE outside the room.

👋 **ALERT:** Be aware that protective precautions are frequently required in the intensive care nursery.

SAFETY

Blood and Body Fluid Cleanup

The disinfectant most commonly used for cleaning blood and body fluid spills in the laboratory is 1:10 sodium hypochlorite (bleach).

- Always wear gloves.
- Absorb the spill with paper towels and discard towels in a biohazard container.
- Cover the spill area with disinfectant and allow the disinfectant to dry.
- A blood spill kit may be available in the area for use.

Sharps Precautions

Ways to Avoid Accidental Needle Punctures

- Never recap a needle.

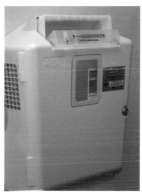

- Activate safety shields immediately after withdrawing the needle.
- Discard needles with the holder attached. Never remove the needle from the holder.
- Always become thoroughly proficient with the operation of new safety devices before using them to draw blood from patients.
- Never reach into a sharps container.

💧 ALERT: Remember that sharps containers should be filled only to the designated mark and NEVER overfilled.

Blood and Body Fluid Exposure Evaluation

Postexposure Protocol
💧 ALERT: Immediately report all possible bloodborne pathogen exposures to your supervisor or employee health department.

1. Draw a baseline blood specimen and test it for HBV, hepatitis C virus (HCV), and human immunodeficiency virus (HIV).
2. If possible, identify the source patient; collect a blood specimen; and test it for HBV, HCV, and HIV. (Be aware that patients must usually give informed consent for these tests, and the results do not become a part of the patient's record. In some states, a physician's order or court order can replace patient consent because a needlestick is considered a significant exposure.)

💧 ALERT: Complete testing within 24 hours for maximum benefit from postexposure prophylaxis (PEP).

Postexposure Prophylaxis

Source Patient Tests Positive for HBV
1. Unvaccinated employees can be given hepatitis B immune globulin and HBV vaccine.
2. Vaccinated employees are tested for immunity and receive PEP, if necessary.

Source Patient Tests Positive for HCV
1. No PEP is recommended.
2. Employee is monitored for early detection of HCV infection and treated appropriately.

Source Patient Tests Positive for HIV
1. Employee is counseled about receiving PEP using zidovudine and one or two additional anti-HIV medications.
2. Medications are started within 24 hours.
3. Employee is retested at intervals of 6 weeks, 12 weeks, and 6 months.
4. Additional evaluation and counseling are needed if the source patient is unidentified or untested.

🖐 **ALERT:** Even if tests are negative, an exposed employee should be counseled to report any symptoms related to viral infection that occur within 12 weeks of the exposure.

SUMMARY OF TRANSMISSION PREVENTION GUIDELINES FOR BLOOD COLLECTORS

- Wear appropriate PPE.
- Change gloves between patients.
- Sanitize hands after removing gloves.
- Dispose of biohazardous material in designated containers.
- Activate the needle safety device before disposing of sharps in sharps containers.
- Properly dispose of sharps in puncture-resistant containers.
- Do not recap needles.
- Do not activate a needle safety device using both hands.
- Follow your facility's protocol governing working during personal illness.
- Maintain personal immunizations.
- Decontaminate work areas and equipment.
- Do not centrifuge uncapped tubes.
- Do not eat, drink, smoke, or apply cosmetics in the work area.

Chemical Precautions

- Take precautions to avoid getting chemicals on the body, clothes, and work area, including:
  - Wearing proper protective clothing.
  - Using corrective chemical cleanup materials.
  - Storing chemicals properly.
- Label containers and never store chemicals in unlabeled containers.
- Carefully follow instructions when mixing chemicals.

✋ ALERT: Never add water to acid.

- Immediately flush the skin and eyes with water for at least 15 minutes whenever contact with acid occurs.

✋ ALERT: Be aware that a Safety Data Sheet (SDS) must be made available to employees for all chemicals containing hazardous ingredients greater than 1%.

Radiation Precautions

All blood collectors can be exposed to radiation while drawing blood from patients in the radiation department, from patients receiving radioactive treatments, and in the laboratory when procedures requiring radioisotopes are used.

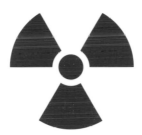

RADIATION

✋ **ALERT:** Blood collectors who are pregnant should avoid areas where this symbol is displayed.

Electrical Precautions

- When drawing blood and performing other procedures, avoid contact with electrical equipment in the patient's room because current from improperly grounded equipment can pass through the blood collector and metal needle to the patient.
- Do not operate electrical equipment with wet hands or while in contact with water.

In Case of Electrical Shock

✋ ALERT: Do not touch the person.

- Turn off the circuit breaker.
- Remove the source equipment using a nonconductive glass or wooden object.
- Get medical assistance.

Fire and Explosion Precautions

Discovery of a Fire

RACE
- **R**escue: Rescue anyone in immediate danger.
- **A**larm: Activate the facility's fire alarm system.
- **C**ontain: Close all doors to potentially affected areas.
- **E**xtinguish/Evacuate: Extinguish the fire, if possible, or evacuate, closing the door behind you.

Operation of a Fire Extinguisher

PASS
- **P**ull pin.
- **A**im at base of fire.
- **S**queeze handles.
- **S**weep nozzle from side to side.

Physical Precautions

- Avoid running in rooms and hallways.
- Be alert for wet floors.
- Bend at the knees when lifting heavy objects or patients.
- Keep long hair tied back and remove dangling jewelry to avoid contact with equipment and patients.
- Wear comfortable, closed-toe shoes with nonskid soles that provide maximum support.
- Maintain a clean, organized work area.

Location of Safety Equipment

Equipment	Workplace 1	Workplace 2
Fire alarm		
Fire extinguisher		
Emergency exit		
Shower		
Eyewash station		
Electrical panel		
First aid kit		
SDS		

Common Laboratory Tests and Collection Tube Requirements

Test	Collection Tube	Comments	Dept.
Acid phosphatase	Serum (red or gold) gel barrier tube	Freeze serum	C
Adrenocorticotropic hormone (ACTH)	Lavender, siliconized glass or plastic	Freeze plasma	C
Alanine aminotransferase (ALT)	Plasma (green) or serum (red or gold) gel barrier tube		C
Albumin	Plasma (green) or serum (red or gold) gel barrier tube		C
Aldosterone	Red	Patient should be lying down for at least 30 minutes before blood collection	C
Alkaline phosphatase (ALP)	Plasma (green) or serum (red or gold) gel barrier tube		C
Alpha-fetoprotein (AFP)	Serum (red or gold) gel barrier tube		C
Aluminum (Al)	Plain royal blue	Do not use gel	C

Continued

Test	Collection Tube	Comments	Dept.
Ammonia (NH_3)	Lavender or green	Send in an ice slurry	C
Amylase	Plasma (green) or serum (red or gold) gel barrier tube		C
Angiotensin-converting enzyme (ACE)	Serum (red or gold) gel barrier tube; red	Place in an ice slurry	C
Antibiotic assays (amikacin, gentamicin, theophylline, tobramycin, vancomycin)	Red; clear non-gel microcollection tube	No gel barrier tubes	C
Antibody identification (ID)/screen	Lavender or pink		BB
Antidiuretic hormone (ADH)	Lavender	Freeze plasma	C
Anti-hepatitis A virus	Serum (red or gold) gel barrier tube; red		C
Anti-hepatitis B surface antigen	Serum (red or gold) gel barrier tube; red		I
Anti-hepatitis C virus	Serum (red or gold) gel barrier tube; red		I
Anti-HIV	Red		I

Continued

Test	Collection Tube	Comments	Dept.
Antinuclear antibody (ANA)	Serum (red or gold) gel barrier tube; red		I
Antistreptolysin O (ASO) titer	Red	Refrigerate immediately or freeze serum	I
Antithrombin III	Light blue	Freeze plasma immediately	CO
Apo-A, Apo-B lipoprotein	Serum (red or gold) gel barrier tube		C
Aspartate aminotransferase (AST)	Plasma (green) or serum (red or gold) gel barrier tube		C
Basic metabolic panel (BMP)	Plasma (green) or serum (red or gold) gel barrier tube		C
Beta human chorionic gonadotropin (beta hCG)	Plasma (green) or serum (red or gold) gel barrier tube		C
Bilirubin, total and direct (Bili)	Plasma (green) or serum (red or gold) gel barrier tube; amber or green microcollection tube	Protect from light	C

Continued

Test	Collection Tube	Comments	Dept.
Blood culture	Blood culture bottles (two bottles, aerobic and anaerobic) or two yellow SPS tubes	Aseptic technique; do not refrigerate	M
Blood group and type (ABO and Rh)	Lavender or pink	Blood bank ID	BB
Blood urea nitrogen (BUN)	Plasma (green) or serum (red or gold) gel barrier tube		C
Brain natriuretic peptide (BNP)	Lavender; white plasma preparation tube; serum gel (red or gold) barrier tube		C
C-peptide	Serum (red or gold; gel barrier tube; red	Stable for 4 hours	C
Calcitonin	Red	Ensure patient has fasted; avoid hemolysis	C
Calcium	Plasma (green) or serum (red or gold) gel barrier tube	No gel barrier tubes; freeze serum immediately	C
		Deliver to the laboratory immediately; refrigerate	C

Continued

Test	Collection Tube	Comments	Dept.
Cancer antigen (CA-125)	Serum (red or gold) gel barrier tube; red	Refrigerate	C
Carbamazepine (Tegretol)	Red	No gel barrier tubes	C
Carbon monoxide (CO)	Lavender; green	Do not underfill; refrigerate immediately	C
Carcinoembryonic antigen (CEA)	Serum (red or gold) gel barrier tube		C
Carotene, beta	Serum (red or gold) gel barrier tube; red	Protect from light	C
Chemistry panels (cardiac, hepatic, metabolic, and renal)	Plasma (green) or serum (red or gold) gel barrier tube		C
Cholesterol	Plasma (green) or serum (red or gold) gel barrier tube		C
Chromium (Cr)	Plain royal blue; EDTA royal blue	Separate and refrigerate immediately	C
Cold agglutinins	Red	Must be kept at 37°C; no gel barrier tubes	I
Comprehensive metabolic panel (CMP)	Plasma (green) or serum (red or gold) gel barrier tube		C

Continued

Test	Collection Tube	Comments	Dept.
Complement levels	Serum (red or gold) gel barrier tube		C
Complete blood count (CBC)	Lavender		H
Copper	Serum royal blue		C
Cortisol	Serum (red or gold) gel barrier tube; red		C
Creatine kinase (CK)	Plasma (green) or serum (red or gold) gel barrier tube	Serum only, timed specimen (a.m.)	C
Creatine kinase isoenzymes (CK-MB, CK-MM, CK-BB)	Serum (red or gold) gel barrier tube		C
Creatinine (Creat)	Plasma (green) or serum (red or gold) gel barrier tube		C
C-reactive protein	Serum (red or gold) or plasma (green) gel barrier tube; red		C
Crossmatch	Lavender; pink	Blood bank ID remains on 72 hours	BB
Cryoglobulin	Red; lavender	Collect in prewarmed tube and keep at 37°C	C

Test	Collection Tube	Comments	Dept.
Cyclosporine	Lavender; green	No gel barrier tubes	C
Differential (Diff)	Lavender	Make blood smear within 1 hour of collection	H
Digoxin	Plasma (green) or serum (red or gold) gel barrier tube; red		C
D-Dimer (D-DI)	Light blue	Tube must be full (stable for 4 hours)	CO
Direct antihuman globulin test (DAT) or direct Coombs	Lavender		BB
Disseminated intravascular coagulation (DIC) panel	Light blue		CO
Drug screen	Red	No gel barrier tubes	C
Electrolytes (Lytes) Na, K, Cl, CO₂	Plasma (green) or serum (red or gold) gel barrier tube	Do not refrigerate specimen	C
Epstein-Barr virus panel	Serum (red or gold) gel barrier tube; red		I
Erythrocyte sedimentation rate (ESR)	Lavender	Tube must be filled at least half-full	H

Continued

Test	Collection Tube	Comments	Dept.
Ethanol/alcohol (ETOH)	Gray	Do not open tube until testing; may require chain of custody; only use nonalcohol solution for skin cleansing	C
Factor assays	Light blue	Tube must be full	C
Fasting blood sugar (FBS)	Plasma (green) or serum (red or gold) gel barrier tube; gray; lavender	Ensure patient has fasted for 8 hours before blood collection	C
Febrile antibody panel	Red		I
Ferritin	Plasma (green) or serum (red or gold) gel barrier tube		C
Fibrin degradation product (FDP)	Special navy blue tube with thrombin	Tube will only fill to 2 mL and should clot immediately	CO
Fibrinogen	Light blue	Tube must be full	C
Fluorescent antinuclear antibody (FANA)	Serum (red or gold) gel barrier tube; red		I

Continued

Test	Collection Tube	Comments	Dept.
Fluorescent treponemal antibody-absorption (FTA-ABS)	Serum (red or gold) gel barrier tube; red		I
Folate	Serum (red or gold) gel barrier tube; red		C
Gamma-glutamyl transpeptidase (GGT)	Serum (red or gold) gel barrier tube; red		C
Gastrin	Serum (red or gold) gel barrier tube	Transport in an ice slurry	C
Glucose-6-phosphate dehydrogenase (G6PD)	Lavender		H
Glucose	Plasma (green) or serum (red or gold) gel barrier tube; red; gray; lavender		C
Hematocrit (Hct)	Lavender		H
Hemoglobin (Hgb)	Lavender		H
Hemoglobin A1c	Lavender		C
Hemoglobin electrophoresis	Lavender		C

Continued

Test	Collection Tube	Comments	Dept.
Hemoglobin/hematocrit (H&H); Hgb/Hct	Lavender		H
Heparin anti-X_a assay	Light blue		CO
Hepatitis B core antibody	Serum (red or gold) gel barrier tube; red		I
Hepatitis B surface antibody	Serum (red or gold) gel barrier tube; red		I
Hepatitis B surface antigen	Serum (red or gold) gel barrier tube; red		I
Homocysteine (Hcy)	Lavender; serum (red or gold) gel barrier tube; red	Place in an ice slurry	C
Human chorionic gonadotropin (hCG)	Plasma (green) or serum (red or gold) gel barrier tube		C
Immunoglobulin levels	Plasma (green) or serum (red or gold) gel barrier tube; red		C
International normalized ratio (INR)	Light blue	Tube must be full	CO
Insulin	Serum (red or gold) gel barrier tube		C

Continued

Test	Collection Tube	Comments	Dept.
Ionized calcium (iCA^{2+})	Serum (red or gold) gel barrier tube; red; arterial blood gas syringe	Tube must be full	C
Iron	Plasma (green) or serum (red or gold) gel barrier tube		C
Iron-binding capacity	Plasma (green) or serum (red or gold) gel barrier tube		C
Lactate dehydrogenase (LD)	Plasma (green) or serum (red or gold) gel barrier tube		C
Lactate (lactic acid) (Lact)	Gray; arterial blood gas syringe	Analyze in 15 minutes; draw without tourniquet; place in an ice slurry when collecting in an arterial blood gas syringe; however, follow facility protocol	C
Lead (Pb)	Royal blue EDTA; tan EDTA; lavender microcollection tube		C
Lipase	Plasma (green) or serum (red or gold) gel barrier tube; red		C

Continued

Test	Collection Tube	Comments	Dept.
Lipoproteins (high-density lipoprotein [HDL], low-density lipoprotein [LDL], very-low density lipoprotein [VLDL])	Plasma (green) or serum (red or gold) gel barrier tube		C
Lithium (Li)	Serum (red or gold) gel barrier tube; red	Drew 12 hours post dose	C
Magnesium	Serum (red or gold) gel barrier tube; red		C
MI panel (CK isoenzyme (CK-MB), myoglobin (Myo), troponin (Tn)	Plasma (green) gel barrier tube; serum (red or gold) gel barrier tube; white plasma preparation tube; lavender	Stable for 4 hours	C
Mono nucleosis screen (Mono test)	Serum (red or gold) gel barrier tube; red		I
Myoglobin	Serum (red or gold) gel barrier tube; red		C
Osmolality	Serum (red or gold) gel barrier tube; red		C
Parathyroid hormone (PTH)	Lavender	Place in an ice slurry	C

Continued

Test	Collection Tube	Comments	Dept.
Partial thromboplastin time (PTT); activated partial thromboplastin time (APTT)	Light blue	Full tube; nonheparinized specimens are stable at RT up to 4 hours; heparinized specimens must be centrifuged within 1 hour and are stable up to 4 hours	CO
pH	Green; non-gel	Send on ice slurry	C
Phosphorus	Plasma (green) or serum (red or gold) gel barrier tube		C
Plasminogen	Light blue	Freeze plasma immediately	CO
Platelet (Plt) aggregation	Light blue and lavender		H
Platelet (Plt)	Lavender		H
Porphyrins	Plasma (green) gel barrier tube	Protect from light	C
Potassium	Plasma (green) or serum (red or gold) gel barrier tube; red		C

Continued

Test	Collection Tube	Comments	Dept.
Prostate-specific antigen (PSA)	Serum (red or gold) gel barrier tube		C
Prostatic acid phosphatase (PAP)	Serum (red or gold) gel barrier tube		C
Protein	Serum (red or gold) gel barrier tube		C
Protein electrophoresis	Serum (red or gold) gel barrier tube; red		C
Prothrombin time (PT)	Light blue	Full tube; stable at RT up to 24 hours	CO
Quantitative protein assay (C3, C4, Immunoglobulins [IgG, IgA, IgM], haptoglobin)	Plasma (green) or serum (red or gold) gel barrier tube; red		I
Rapid plasmin reagin (RPR)	Serum (red or gold) gel barrier tube; red		I
Red blood cell (RBC) count	Lavender		H
Reticulocyte count (Retic)	Lavender		H
Rheumatoid factor (RF)	Serum (red or gold) gel barrier tube; red		I

Continued

Test	Collection Tube	Comments	Dept.
Rubella titer	Serum (red or gold) gel barrier tube; red		I
Salicylate (aspirin)	Red	No gel barrier tubes	C
Sickle cell screening	Lavender		H
Sodium	Plasma (green) or serum (red or gold) gel barrier tube; red		C
T-cell count	Lavender		I
Testosterone	Serum (red or gold) gel barrier tube		C
Therapeutic drugs (digoxin, theophylline [theo], phenobarbital, phenytoin [Phenyl], carbamazepine [Carb], valproic acid [val ac])	Red; clear non-gel microcollection tube	No gel barrier tubes; centrifuge and separate within 1 hour	C
Thyroid-stimulating hormone/Free T$_4$ (TSH/T$_4$)	Plasma (green) or serum (red or gold) gel barrier tube		C
Total protein (TP)	Serum (red or gold) gel barrier tube		C

Continued

Test	Collection Tube	Comments	Dept.
Triglycerides	Plasma (green) or serum (red or gold) gel barrier tube		C
Troponin I and T	Serum (red or gold) gel barrier tube; lavender; white plasma preparation tube		C
Type and screen	Lavender/pink	Blood bank ID	BB
Uric acid	Serum (red or gold) gel barrier tube		C
Valproic acid (Depakote)	Red	No gel barrier tubes	C
Venereal Disease Research Laboratory (VDRL)	Serum (red or gold) gel barrier tube; red		I
Viral load	Lavender; white plasma preparation tube; serum (red or gold) gel barrier tube	Freeze plasma immediately	I
Vitamin A	Red	No gel barrier tubes; ensure patient has fasted	C

Continued

CLSI Recommended Order of Draw

Order	Tube Color	Additive	Number of Inversions
1	Yellow	SPS Sterile media bottles	8–10
2	Light blue	Sodium citrate	3–4
3	Red plastic	Clot activator	5
	Red glass	No additive	0
	Red and gray SST	Gel separator tube with clot activator	5
	Gold SST	Gel separator tube with clot activator	5
	Orange RST	Gel separator tube with thrombin	5–6
	Royal blue	Clot activator	5–6
4	Light green PST	Gel separator tube with heparin	8–10
	Green	Heparin	
	Royal blue	Heparin	
5	Lavender	EDTA	8–10
	Pink	EDTA	
	Tan	EDTA	
	Royal blue	EDTA	
	White PPT	Gel separator with EDTA	
6	Gray	Potassium oxalate Sodium fluoride	8–10
7	Yellow	ACD	8–10

Courtesy of © Becton, Dickinson and Company. Adapted with permission.

Phlebotomy Notes
Pocket Guide to Blood Collection
SECOND EDITION

Your go-to guide for the must-know information you need to collect, transport, and process specimens safely and effectively.

★ ★ ★ ★ ★ **Awesome.** *"I have referred all my classmates to purchase this excellent resource. Even my instructor was impressed with it. You will not find a more handy and complete pocket guide."*

★ ★ ★ ★ ★ **If you're studying phlebotomy, you NEED this!** *"One word...Excellent!"*

★ ★ ★ ★ ★ **Jam-packed with information.** *"This is an excellent product to have for phlebotomy. It has an enormous amount of information that was very helpful in studying to pass the exam and will be great to have on the job. Highly recommend."*

—Amazon Review

Must-have information—to go

Look for more Davis's Notes online at FADavis.com

F.A. DAVIS
Independent Publishers Since 1879
FADavis.com

ISBN 978-0-8036...

9 780803 6...

P9-CTJ-966

Inches

Centimeters

Dermal Puncture Sites

Dermal puncture is the method of choice for collecting blood from infants and children younger than 2 years and for adults with inaccessible or fragile veins.

Heel (for Infants Younger Than Age 1 Year)
■ Use the medial and lateral areas of the bottom (plantar) surface.

Heel Puncture Sites

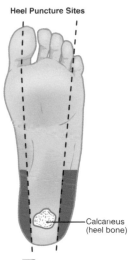

Calcaneus
(heel bone)

 Puncture zone

👆 ALERT: Do not puncture the posterior aspect of the heel.

DERMAL
PUNCT

DERMAL PUNCT

Finger (for Adults and Children Older Than Age 1 Year)

■ Use the fleshy area located between the center and the lateral side of the third or fourth finger on the palmar side.

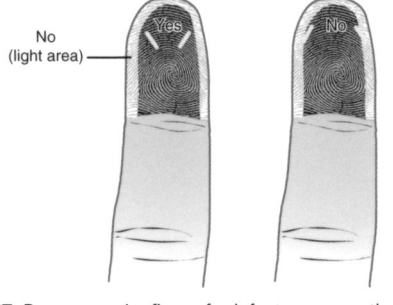

No
(light area)

Yes

No

👆 **ALERT:** Do not use the finger for infants younger than age 1 year.

SITES TO AVOID

■ Back of the heel
■ Arch of the foot
■ Previously used sites
■ Areas with visible damage
■ Swollen sites
■ Earlobes
■ Fingers on the side of a mastectomy

Dermal Puncture Procedure

Equipment

- Requisition form
- Gloves
- 70% isopropyl alcohol pads
- Finger or heel puncture device

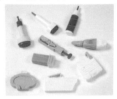

- 2-inch × 2-inch gauze
- Warming device
- Sharps disposal container
- Indelible pen
- Bandage
- Biohazard bag
- Microcollection tube or capillary tubes

✋ **ALERT:** Microcollection tubes are color-coded to match evacuated tube colors and include amber-colored tubes for light-sensitive analyte testing.

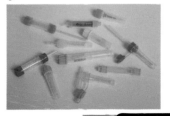

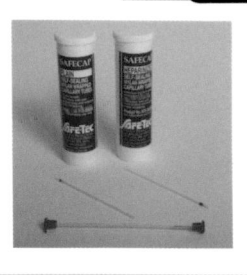

Procedure

1. Obtain and examine the requisition form. Check for completeness, date and time of collection, and priority.
2. Greet the patient, and explain the procedure.
3. Identify the patient using two identifiers. Ask a parent or guardian to identify an infant or a child or compare the ID band with the requisition form.
4. Verify adherence to dietary and medication restrictions.
5. Ask about latex allergies and previous problems with blood collection.
6. Position the patient:
   - For a heelstick, position the infant on his or her back with the foot lower than the body.
   - For a fingerstick, position the patient's arm on a firm surface with the hand palm up and fingers pointing downward.
7. Select the proper equipment according to the patient's age, type of test ordered, and amount of blood to be collected.

👆 **ALERT:** Follow the manufacturer's directions for selection of puncture device. The type of device used depends on the age of the patient, amount of blood required, collection site, and puncture depth.

8. Sanitize your hands using the proper technique.
9. Apply gloves, and put on a gown if required by the nursery.

119

ALERT: Turn off an ultraviolet light (bili light) when collecting specimens for newborn bilirubin tests.

10. Select the puncture site.
11. For optimal blood flow, warm the area to be punctured either by:
    - Placing a towel that has been moistened with warm water (42°C) on the site (requires you to dry the site before puncture), or
    - Activating a commercial warmer and covering the site for 3 to 5 minutes.

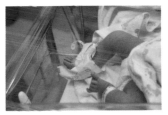

12. Cleanse the site with 70% isopropyl alcohol, and allow it to air-dry.
13. Prepare the lancet by removing the lancet locking device.
14. Open the cap to the microcollection tube.
15. Grasp and position the area to be punctured:
    - For a heelstick, grasp the heel with your index finger around the arch, your thumb around the bottom, and your other fingers around the top of the foot.
    - For a fingerstick, hold the finger between your nondominant thumb and index finger, with the palmar surface facing up and the finger pointing downward.
16. Place the lancet firmly on the fleshy area of the finger or heel perpendicular to the fingerprint or heelprint.

DERMAL PUNCT

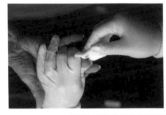

17. Depress the lancet trigger.
18. Discard the lancet in an approved sharps disposal container.

👤 **ALERT:** Failure to place the puncture device firmly on the skin is the primary cause of insufficient blood flow.

19. Gently squeeze the finger or heel.
20. Wipe away the first drop of blood because it may contain alcohol residue and tissue fluid.

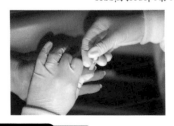

21. Collect rounded drops into the appropriate collection device:
   ▪ Gently apply pressure to and release pressure from the area. Do not milk the site or surrounding tissue.

👋 **ALERT**: Applying pressure about 1 inch away from the puncture site frequently produces better blood flow than applying pressure very close to the site.

- For microcollection tubes:
  - Place the tip of the collection tube beneath the puncture site and touch the underside of the drop.

👋 **ALERT**: Do not scrape the skin while collecting the specimen.

  - Slant the tube downward during collection to allow blood to run through the capillary collection scoop and down the side of the tube.
  - If necessary, gently tap the bottom of the tube to force the blood to the bottom.
  - Cap each microcollection tube when the correct amount of blood has been collected.

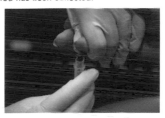

- For microhematocrit tubes:
  - Place the end of a microhematocrit tube into the drop of blood.
  - Maintain the tube in a horizontal position to fill by capillary action during the entire collection.
  - When the tubes are filled, seal them with sealant clay.

👆 **ALERT**: Collect the specimen within 2 minutes to prevent clotting.

22. Collect in the correct **order of draw**:
    - Capillary blood gases
    - Blood smear
    - Microhematocrit capillary tubes
    - Lavender EDTA microcollection tubes
    - Other anticoagulated microcollection tubes
    - Serum microcollection tubes

👆 **ALERT**: Remember that dermal puncture order of draw differs from venipuncture order of draw.

23. After capping or sealing the tubes, mix them by gently inverting them 5 to 10 times.
24. Place gauze on the site, and apply pressure until the bleeding stops.
25. Label the tubes before leaving the patient, and verify identification with the patient.
26. Examine the site for bleeding cessation.
27. Apply a bandage if the patient is older than 2 years.
28. Dispose of used supplies in biohazard containers.
29. Thank the patient.
30. Remove your gloves.
31. Sanitize your hands.
32. Prepare the specimen and requisition form for transportation to the laboratory, making sure to observe special handling instructions.

Order of Draw Using BD Microtainer Tubes

Microguard™ Closure	Additive	Inv.	Laboratory Use
Lavender	K_2 EDTA	10x	For whole blood hematology determinations. Tube inversions prevent clotting.
Green	Lithium Heparin	10x	For plasma determinations in chemistry. Tube inversions prevent clotting.
Mint Green	Lithium Heparin and Gel for plasma separation	10x	For plasma determinations in chemistry. Tube inversions prevent clotting. Available in clear and amber-colored tubes.
Gray	NaFl/Na_2 EDTA	10x	For glucose determinations. Tube inversions ensure proper mixing of additive and blood.
Gold	Clot Activator and Gel for serum separation	5x	For serum determinations in chemistry. Available in clear and amber-colored tubes.
Red	No additive	0x	For serum determinations in chemistry, serology, and blood banking.

Inv. = Inversion

DERMAL PUNCT

Dermal Puncture Notes